An Evidence Base for Ophthalmic Nursing Practice

Edited by Janet Marsden
Manchester Metropolitan University

D1428492

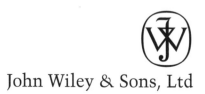

John Wiley & Sons, Ltd

Other Wiley Editorial Offices

John Wiley & Sons Inc., 111 River Street, Hoboken, NJ 07030, USA

Jossey-Bass, 989 Market Street, San Francisco, CA 94103-1741, USA

Wiley-VCH Verlag GmbH, Boschstr. 12, D-69469 Weinheim, Germany

John Wiley & Sons Australia Ltd, 42 McDougall Street, Milton, Queensland 4064, Australia

John Wiley & Sons (Asia) Pte Ltd, 2 Clementi Loop #02-01, Jin Xing Distripark, Singapore
129809

John Wily & Sons Canada Ltd, 6045 Freemont Blvd, Mississauga, ONT, L5R 4J3, Canada

Wiley also publishes its books in a variety of electronic formats. Some content that appears in
print may not be available in electronic books.

Library of Congress Cataloging-in-Publication Data

An evidence base for ophthalmic nursing practice / edited by Janet Marsden.
    p. ; cm.
  Includes bibliographical references and index.
  ISBN 978-0-470-05798-8 (pbk.)
1. Ophthalmic nursing. 2. Evidence-based nursing. I. Marsden, Janet.
  [DNLM: 1. Eye Diseases–nursing. 2. Ophthalmology–methods. 3. Evidence-Based
Medicine–methods.   WY 158 E93 2007]
  RE88.E38 2007
  617.7'0231–dc22

                                                                    2007034312

British Library Cataloguing in Publication Data

A catalogue record for this book is available from the British Library

ISBN   9780470057988

Set in 9/11 pt Palatino by SNP Best-set Typesetter Ltd., Hong Kong
Printed and bound in Singapore by Markono Print Media Pte Ltd

This book is printed on acid-free paper responsibly manufactured from sustainable forestry
in which at least two trees are planted for each one used for paper production.

Contents

Contents

Contents

Preface

The evidence base for ophthalmic care is often scanty. Practice differs, with different rationales in different areas and, often, we do not really know why we do what we do. This book was born out of the recognition by the Royal College of Nursing's Ophthalmic Nursing Forum Steering Committee that best practice in ophthalmic care across the UK should be synthesised along with the evidence to support it, to enable practitioners to develop guidelines and to identify and use the best evidence possible in the care of patients with ophthalmic problems.

This book aims to address some of these issues. Where there is robust evidence, it is identified, practitioner experience is incorporated and, when there is no obvious 'scientific' evidence, consensus expert opinion is included.

In many ways, this is 'work in progress'. Practice will continue to evolve; we will get more effective at both synthesising evidence and actually researching our own practice. Evidence will be found to support, and refute, our work and we must be open minded enough to debate issues around practice and to change when we need to. More topics will need to be considered as new techniques and therapies are developed.

We hope that this book is useful and if there is any progress or evidence that you want to let us know about, do please contact me.

Janet Marsden
j.marsden@mmu.ac.uk
June 2007

Contributors

Stephen Craig, Senior Lecturer, Northumbria University

Helen Davies, Lead Nurse, Ophthalmology, HM Stanley Hospital, St Asaph

Janet Marsden, Senior Lecturer, Manchester Metropolitan University

Joan Mathison, Nurse Practitioner, Princess Alexandra Eye Pavilion, Edinburgh

Yvonne Needham, Head of Pre-registration, Nurse Education, The University of Hull

Jenny Nosek, Sister, Ophthalmology, Royal Wolverhampton Hospitals NHS Trust

Mary Shaw, Senior Lecturer (teaching), The University of Manchester

Nicky Shute, Senior Clinical Nurse, Queen Mary's Hospital, Sidcup

Mary Stott, Sister, Ophthalmology, Royal Wolverhampton Hospitals NHS Trust

Sandra Taylor, Nurse Manager/AMD Research Study Coordinator, St Paul's Clinical Eye Research Centre, Royal Liverpool University Hospital

Julie Tillotson, Advanced Nurse Practitioner, Bournemouth Eye Unit

Introduction: evidence and practice

This book considers some of the evidence base for ophthalmic nursing practice – the 'whys' of what we do. My interest in the evidence base for practice began fairly early in my nursing career when I realised that, often, there was little obvious reason for why we did what we did and when I asked why (because I'm like that!) no one could really explain. One of my first forays into using actual evidence in practice was after I read somewhere that EUSOL (Edinburgh University Solution of Lime for those readers who are old enough to remember), a wound cleaning solution that appeared to work very well, stopped tissue granulation. It cleaned the wound beautifully, but damaged the wound bed and actually resulted in a clean wound, although one that healed poorly. The evidence was very persuasive and chimed with my own experience, so the nurses in the department that I was managing at the time discussed changing our practice – and stopped using it, much to the disgust of our medical colleagues! Over the years, I have become even more interested (not to say a little obsessive about asking 'why?') and hope that this book helps to provide some of the answers. It has been prepared by a team of nurses who are passionate about their speciality – past and present members of the steering committee of the Ophthalmic Nursing Forum of the Royal College of Nursing.

WHAT IS EVIDENCE-BASED PRACTICE?

First of all, it is not hearsay – 'I heard this was true so we must do it' is not a good basis for practice. Nor is it the result of a single (bad) paper. It is interesting that sometimes a single notion can 'change the world' of work. An example of this was in 1998 when a single paper, published in the *British Medical Journal*, suggested that topical chloramphenicol, one of our mainstays of treatment and a prophylaxis for ophthalmic infection, had the same effect as the systemic drug and could precipitate blood dyscrasias, including aplastic anaemia (Lancaster et al. 1998). Despite a robust refutation of this (Walker et al. 1998), almost all the general accident and emergency departments in the UK appeared to stop using this drug immediately (most doctors appear to read the *BMJ* if nothing else; the second paper was in *Eye* – a specifically ophthalmic journal – it really matters where you publish your evidence!). Ophthalmology, in general, ignored the available 'evidence' and did not alter practice. Subsequently, the results of Lancaster's paper have been discredited and it is now generally believed that topical chloramphenicol is extremely safe (Field et al. 1999) and is widely used in both general and ophthalmic emergency departments.

Evidence-based practice is not what you're told to do – following orders has never been a good defence for inappropriate action! Our profession needs nurses who say why – incessantly – and are not happy until they get a good answer!

It is not what we have always done either – stagnation results when we continue to do what we have always done. The many and varied rituals in nursing seem to be gradually diminishing but I am sure that many remain.

Evidence-based practice is a careful consideration of all the information available and a decision based on this, and the particular situation in which the clinician and patient find themselves.

WHAT IS EVIDENCE?

How do we know what we know? Knowledge can be classified in a number of ways such as:

- Experiential knowledge: such as how to swim or ride a bicycle; the things we learn by experience that will always be part of what we know.
- Mutual knowledge: how we all know that spiders are more frightened of us than we are of them.
- Formal knowledge: the systematic exploration and sifting of evidence.

- Tacit knowledge: that which we do not know we know.
- Craft-based knowledge: that which goes with the job.
- Common knowledge: that which we all know.

In 'civilian' and professional life we use all these types of knowledge and in nursing we use combinations of these. This becomes our nursing knowledge, which in turn informs our practice. There has to be a balance between these types of knowledge in our work, however, and we must 'evidence' what we do with formal or scientific knowledge so that our practice is based on evidence, rather than myth and tradition. We must be aware of the evidence that informs our experience, and if there is not any, perhaps we need to think about how we can go about producing some.

There are many different types of evidence that may inform practice: scientific knowledge may be in the form of international, national or more local research. Meta-analysis and systematic reviews are said to constitute the highest level of evidence because they synthesise all the available evidence; however, minor decisions and differences in the literature-searching and review process can have a major impact on the results. Meta-analyses may be compromised by the scales chosen (and there are many) to rate and therefore select the evidence to be analysed. Large, international and national research studies may be felt to be at a high level within any hierarchy of evidence. They are likely to be high-quality research but, as with any research, must be read with a critical eye. They may not, although generalisable in theory, give the answers that you need in your particular practice. The funding for large-scale research often follows health priorities and the area that you are interested in may not, at present, be a priority area. The evidence may therefore not be available when you need it. Local research evidence uses small-scale studies to investigate local problems and, although not necessarily generalisable to large populations, may be useful in your particular practice and available (or do-able) when you need it. There is no reason why small studies should not be just as rigorous as large studies are (or are intended to be) and often have much more relevance to local patient populations.

Other evidence that is available includes consensus and expert opinion and this is often available in your local area – your clinical experience and that of other clinicians around you is often very valuable and should not be discarded, as long as objectivity is maintained and biases are identified!

This informal knowledge is often context specific, and all clinicians must be aware that it needs continual review and updating. Never forget though that as Neils Bohr (a Danish physicist) said, 'An expert is someone who has made all the mistakes that can be made, but in a very narrow field' (Bohr, quoted in Mackay 1994).

Ultimately, evidence is knowledge of varying types, from a variety of different sources. The claims made for it must be commensurate with the strength of the evidence and for local use and within a given context; informal knowledge is often both adequate and effective. For wider application, or for situations of potential major impact, stronger evidence is required. Where robust research evidence does not exist (and in many areas, it would be unethical to start trying to prove why we do what we do, because we have been doing it for so long that it has become normal practice), expert and, even better, consensus-based expert opinion is the best evidence available.

WHAT DO WE DO ONCE WE HAVE EVIDENCE?
The two main things that need to be done with available evidence are evaluation and application.

Evaluation

To evaluate the evidence clinicians need the ability to analyse the evidence critically – to read more than just the abstract, or the introduction and conclusion of an academic article, and to understand it (and sometimes this can take a while!). The ability to analyse evidence critically is not enough on its own though. Evidence must relate to practice and must be critiqued, when it is to be applied in practice, through a filter of subject expertise.

Application

An example of this might be: why do ophthalmic professionals often give an antibiotic ointment if a patient has corneal epithelial loss? Evidence shows that ointment may actually retard epithelial healing and there is no large study that compares antibiotic with no antibiotic and looks at healing. It could be suggested, therefore, that antibiotic and ointment are not required. However, our ophthalmic subject expertise tells us that the tight junctions of corneal epithelium stop pathogen ingress into corneal tissue and further into the eye. If epithelium is lost, as in corneal foreign body or corneal abrasion, the major defence of the eye against pathogens is reduced. Some pathogens are devastating to the eye, all are difficult to treat if they enter the eye and can result in loss of the eye. We give antibiotics after corneal epithelial loss as a prophylaxis against infection rather than as a healing agent, and as clinicians, we know that the greasy film of ointment between the eye and lid is often more comfortable than just a drop.

APPLICATION OF EVIDENCE IN PRACTICE

To apply evidence in practice, clinical experience is key. Practice is not just about the application of scientific or pseudoscientific rules. Clinical experience, based on personal observation, reflection and judgement, is needed to translate scientific rules into the care of individual patients.

Research generalises and considers probabilities of situations occurring; it may also be situational and not applicable in a particular circumstance. Research evidence may be population based, expressed in terms of probability and risk that are helpful indicators, but the results are not necessarily applicable to an individual – it depends on the individuals being alike or at least interchangeable. Ultimately, patients are individuals; they are all different and the application of evidence should be used to enhance practice, not used as a blanket with which to smother individualised care. Clinical experience is the crucial element that separates evidence-based practice from practice by rote and the mindless application of research-based data and, while experience is often characterised as anecdotal, ungeneralisable and a poor basis on which to make scientific decisions, it is often a more powerful persuader than scientific publication in changing clinical practice. Combining clinical experience with good evidence is the key to what Sackett et al. (1996: 71) say evidence-based medicine, or practice in this case, should be:

> Evidence based medicine is the conscientious, explicit and judicious use of best evidence in making decisions about the care of individual patients.

The question to ask is whether the results or evidence will help me in caring for my patients – often this is not expressed in the literature, or is done in a perfunctory way. To add to our evaluation skills of critical analysis and subject expertise, therefore, we need clinical expertise.

VALUES AND CULTURE

The dominant culture in a particular area may affect how evidence and expertise are valued, for example, a very quantitative culture may downgrade the usefulness of qualitative studies. A very medicalised culture may downplay or denigrate the value and usefulness of nursing or other allied health professions' research. Conversely, quantitative evidence may be discarded because it generalises – or because we do not understand the statistics!

Values are often not recognised but play an important part in the application of evidence. Those who believe in complementary medicine, for example, may highlight any information that supports its use whereas those who do not may ignore any positive evidence.

Practitioners vary in what they regard as reliable evidence; each is influenced by his or her own interests and values, which will affect the way that he or she interprets facts and information; evidence is rarely definitive.

Experience leads to systems of belief – evidence may challenge those beliefs and clinicians may find it very difficult to accept evidence that is counterintuitive for them. Evidence may therefore be ignored. Bleek (2000) proposed a different hierarchy of evidence to what is normally accepted but which perhaps reflects how many people operate (Box 1)!

BOX 1
Class 0 Things that I believe
Class 0a Things that I believe despite the available data
Class 1 Randomised controlled clinical trials that agree with what I believe
Class 2 Other prospectively collected data
Class 3 Expert opinion
Class 4 Randomised controlled clinical trials that don't agree with what I believe
Class 5 What you believe that I don't
From Bleek (2000).

Although this is very tongue in cheek it is not hard to recognise the validity of what Bleek proposes in ourselves and in others. Evidence that supports tends to be accepted more readily than evidence that challenges deeply held values.

FINANCE
Practice is often finance influenced and what is best practice, according to the evidence and the situation in which the clinician and patient find themselves, may not be possible because of its cost or availability. What must be aimed for, in this case, is the best available practice and the least compromise in care, an uncomfortable notion for most clinicians and one that is hard to explain to patients in an era where best practice information is so readily available.

CHANGE
Change is often difficult and uncomfortable and persuasion, tact and other highly developed change management skills are likely to be needed to modify deeply held beliefs. It is always nice to be surprised, however, and it may be that colleagues are ready for change, open to suggestion, eager to try new things and receptive to evidence and the need for it as a basis for practice.

EVIDENCE INTO PRACTICE

To ensure a robust evidence base to our practice therefore, we need to be able to evaluate the evidence using our critical analysis skills and subject expertise. To apply the evidence, we need clinical expertise and an objective stance, along with an awareness of competing ideas and robust change management skills!

And finally, something that I found quite recently, but which demonstrates very effectively an argument for evidence rather than ritual, rumour and gossip:

> Do not believe in anything simply because you have heard it
>
> Do not believe in anything simply because it is spoken and rumoured by many
>
> Do not believe in anything simply because it is found written in your religious books
>
> Do not believe in anything merely on the authority of your teachers and elders
>
> Do not believe in traditions because they have been handed down for many generations
>
> But after observation and analysis, when you find that anything agrees with reason and is conducive to the good and benefit of one and all, then accept it and live up to it. (Gautama Buddha AD 430)

Ultimately, applying evidence in our practice will challenge the way that we work and may be contrary to some of our most deeply held beliefs about nursing and the way that we care for our patients and clients; however, embracing the concept of evidence-based practice means taking on things that you do not like as well as things that you do!

REFERENCES

Bleek TB (2000). Letter. *BMJ* **321**:329.

Field D, Martin D, Witchell L (1999). Ophthalmic chloramphenicol: a review of the literature. *Accident Emerg Nursing* **7**(1):13–17.

Lancaster T, Swart AM, Jick H (1998). Risk of serious haematological toxicity with use of chloramphenicol eye drops in a British general practice database. *BMJ* **316**:667.

Mackay AL (1994). *Dictionary of Scientific Quotations*. London: Institute of Physics Publishing.

Sackett DL, Rosenberg JA, Muir Grey JA, Haynes R Brian, Scott Richardson W (1996). Evidence based medicine: what it is and what it isn't. *BMJ* **312**:71–2.

Walker S, Diaper CJ, Bowman R, Sweeney G (1998). Lack of evidence for systemic toxicity following topical chloramphenicol use. *Eye* **12**(Pt 5):875–9.

Section 1

Lids and lacrimal

Basal cell carcinoma

Basal cell carcinoma (BCC) is a proliferation of the basal cells of the dermis in human skin. There are four recognised types of BCC: nodular, cystic, granular and sclerosing. Nodular BCC is the most common finding and easily recognised with a little experience.

Basal cell carcinomas rarely metastasise but do retain the capacity to do so. Twenty-four per cent of all diagnosed BCCs are to be found in the eyelids and BCCs make up 90% of malignant lid lesions (Sowka et al. 2007). Incorrect diagnosis is possible, with confusions being made with sebaceous cysts, squamous cell carcinomas, solar keratosis and chalazion.

SIGNS AND SYMPTOMS
Typically, all except the sclerosing type have a similar pattern of growth. A discrete spot appears that is not troublesome to the patient. Over a period of 12–18 months the spot slowly grows to 10 mm in diameter. A well-defined, rolled, pearlesque edge is evident. Also present is hyperpigmentation of the lesion, often with small blood vessels growing through it close to the skin surface (telangiectasis).

Nodular and cystic lesions bleed easily and the patient often reports that touching a lesion will produce this effect. Patients often present with a lesion with a bloody crust sitting in the crater at the centre of the BCC.

DIAGNOSIS
Diagnosis is based on careful ophthalmic history taking and inspection of the lesion. The only sure way of confirming diagnosis is by histological analysis. Depending on the site of the lesion a wedge biopsy will be performed, and should include the

centre of the lesion, the edge and a sample of normal skin; this biopsy is sometimes known as a Panttone biopsy. The wedge biopsy confirms the diagnosis but preserves most of the lesion *in situ* and the surrounding skin, for more accurate excision and improved cosmetic outcome.

If the lesion is positioned in such a place, with adequate spare skin, the lesion can be removed in its entirety and the wound sutured. Most BCCs require no further treatment; however, some patients do need adjunctive treatment such as radiotherapy.

All suspicious lid lesions that demonstrate irregular growth, changes in colour or appearance, or purulent or bloody discharge, should be biopsied to rule out cancer (Sowka et al. 2007).

CAUSES

Basal cell carcinomas arise in hair-bearing skin, particularly in the periorbital region. Incidence is more pronounced in the lower lid, medial canthus, upper lid and lateral canthus (Tasman and Jaeger 2002).

Aggravating contributory factors include age, smoking and outdoor occupations. There is no recognised gender difference in incidence. Skin type is also a significant factor with a skin type that 'always burns' being more vulnerable.

TREATMENTS

The vast majority of BCCs can be removed in their entirety during a minor surgical list. Some larger BCCs in some lid areas, particularly medially and in young, tight-skinned patients, should be removed using Mohs' procedure, which involves removing minute areas of the lesion, continually sending sections to histopathology for confirmation of malignancy. This procedure continues until 'clear tissue' is returned and ensures that only the minimum amount of tissue is removed, preserving the maximum amount of normal tissue to ensure wound reconstruction and closure.

LIKELY PROGNOSIS

Prognosis depends upon the duration of the BCC and histopathological data; however, BCCs rarely metastasise (Royal

College of Ophthalmologists: www.rcopth.ac.uk). If the patient requires referral to the oncology services, careful liaison should be ensured between the services to promote a holistic and seamless approach to care and management.

FOLLOW-UP CARE
Follow-up care depends on the treatment options. All lesions are removed surgically and standard postoperative wound care should be managed. Long-term postoperative advice should include gentle massage and moisturisation of the wound. Patients should be advised that there is a greater chance of developing a second and third lesion after having already developed one. Careful inspection of the face during personal hygiene time should be advised. Support of the patient should be considered at the time of diagnosis and discharge. If not adequately supported, patients could go through unreasonable anxiety with a cancer diagnosis and lifelong observation for a recurrence!

PATIENT EDUCATION
Sunblock, especially for the face, should be advised, together with regular inspection of the facial skin for recurrence of a BCC.

Patients must be told that, although a BCC requires prompt treatment, BCCs rarely metastasise and are the most common of skin cancers in the UK. Incidence is approximately 144 per million of the UK population (Wong et al. 2003).

REFERENCES
Sowka JW, Gurwood AS, Kaba AG (2007). Basal cell carcinoma. *Handbook of Ocular Disease Management*. Available at: www.revoptom.com/handbook/sect1e.htm (accessed 1 June 2007).

Tasman W, Jaeger E (2002). *Duane's Clinical Ophthalmology*. New York: Lippincott, Williams & Wilkins.

Wong CSM, Strange RC, Lear JT (2003). Basal cell carcinoma. *BMJ* **327**:794–8.

Blepharitis

Blepharitis is not merely a chronic inflammatory condition affecting the eyelids, because the term 'blepharitis' encompasses a range of inflammatory eyelid conditions. It can be divided into anterior types affecting principally the eyelash follicles and posterior types affecting the meibomian glands. Patients frequently present with a combination of the two. It is often associated with ophthalmic disease such as conjunctivitis, chalazion, trichiasis and dry eye, as well as keratitis.

Blepharitis may be associated with acne rosacea and atopic dermatitis. In such cases the underlying cause should be addressed (Shah et al. 1999).

TREATMENT
It may be symptomatic or asymptomatic and, in either case, treatment is recommended (McQueen 2006).

Management of blepharitis is focused around lid hygiene.

- A solution of boiled, cooled tap water and baby shampoo (1 teaspoon to a mug), and good quality cotton buds are required.
- Advise the patient to scrub the lid margins using a new cotton bud for each eye, twice a day for 2 weeks, followed by the same regimen on alternate days for 2 weeks. To prevent further flare-up, it is advisable to perform lid hygiene once a week.
- An alternative to the cotton bud is a clean facecloth wrapped around a finger. A clean flannel should be used each time.
- Alternative solutions include plain cooled boiled water, which is good where there is sensitivity to other solutions, saline and bicarbonate of soda. The last is efficacious in meibomitis

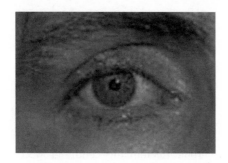

Figure 2.1 Blepharitis.

and where symptoms include burning and itchy sensation (Shah et al. 1999; Shaw 2002; Paranjpe and Foulks 2003; McQueen 2006).

- Where there are shower facilities, the patient should be advised to scrub the eyelids with a clean flannel while showering.

Paranjpe and Foulks (2003) recommend a warm compress and eyelid massage: a clean facecloth soaked in warm water is applied to the closed lids for 2 minutes at a time, followed by massage. The combined action softens the oily secretions and serves to unblock ducts.

In severe cases, as well as this hygiene regimen, oral and topical antibiotics are recommended (Shah et al. 1999).

REFERENCES

McQueen L (2006). Eyelids and lacrimal drainage system. In: Marsden J (ed.), *Ophthalmic Care*. Chichester: Wiley.

Paranjpe DR, Foulks GN (2003). Therapy for meibomian gland disease. *Ophthal Clinics N Am* **16**:37–42.

Shah P, Jacks AS, Khaw PT (1999). *Eye Disease in Clinical Practice*. Rickmansworth: Manticore Europe Ltd.

Shaw ME (2002). Recognising and managing blepharitis. *Int J Ophthal Nursing* **6**:22–5.

Cellulitis

The orbital septum is a layer of fascia extending from the periosteum of the orbital rim to the levator aponeurosis in the upper lid, and then to the inferior border of the tarsal plate in the lower lid. Preseptal cellulitis and orbital cellulitis are major infections of the ocular adnexal and orbital tissues.

PRESEPTAL CELLULITIS

This is an infection of the subcutaneous tissues anterior to the orbital septum. Rapid progression to orbital cellulitis can occur in some patients, especially children. Preseptal cellulitis can be a result of trauma to the skin or infected insect bites. Local infection, such as an infected chalazion or dacryocystitis, may spread to become preseptal cellulitis or a more remote infection such as a middle-ear infection may be transmitted via the blood supply to the lids.

Presentation will be as a unilateral, tender and red periorbital area, with some lid oedema. Treatment is with a course of oral antibiotics such as flucloxacillin or amoxicillin.

ORBITAL CELLULITIS

Orbital cellulitis may follow:

- an infection of the periorbital structures, commonly the paranasal sinuses, but also the face, globe or lacrimal sac
- pathogen ingress after trauma or surgery
- bacteraemia elsewhere through haematogenous spread.

The medial orbital wall is thin and has a number of defects in it (for blood vessels, etc.) allowing for infection to spread to the sub-periorbital space and orbit from the ethmoid sinuses. Venous drainage from the face and paranasal sinuses is mainly via the orbital veins, allowing the passage of infection to the orbits. Ethmoid sinusitis is the most common cause of orbital cellulitis in all age groups.

Orbital cellulitis is more common in winter because of the increased incidence of sinusitis. It is more common in children – their anatomy allows easier passage of infection past the orbital septum from a preseptal cellulitis. In adults, there is no difference in prevalence between the sexes, but, in children, it tends to be more common in boys.

Before the possibility of antibiotic therapy, patients with orbital cellulitis had a mortality rate of 17%, and 20% of survivors were blind in the affected eye. Even with antibiotic therapy, visual loss can result in significant long-term problems (Ferguson and McNab 1999; Harrington 2006).

Orbital cellulitis caused by meticillin-resistant *Staphylococcus aureus* (MRSA) can lead to blindness despite antibiotic treatment (Rutar et al. 2005).

Presenting signs and symptoms (although presentation is variable)

Initially:

- Lid erythema and oedema
- Pain
- A very (dark) red eye
- Conjunctival chemosis
- Fever
- Headache
- Malaise
- History of URTI (upper respiratory tract infection) or sinusitis.

This may progress rapidly to:

- Decreased vision
- Pain on eye movement
- Ophthalmoplegia (reduced eye movement caused by swelling and infection in the orbit and manifesting as diplopia)

- Raised intraocular pressure (IOP)
- Proptosis.

The patient should be asked about recent trauma or dental surgery and he or she, particularly if a child, may be very ill on presentation and the symptoms may get worse very rapidly.

Investigations

Computed tomography (CT) of the orbit and brain is required urgently to evaluate the infection and the degree of spread. Magnetic resonance imaging (MRI) may also be undertaken.

Bloods are normally taken – a full blood screen and, sometimes, blood cultures.

Treatment

The patient should be admitted to hospital and assessed frequently because orbital cellulitis can be vision or even life threatening. Antibiotic regimens differ but usually include intravenous antibiotics, and therapy should be continued until the patient has been fever free for 4 days. Oral antibiotics may continue for variable periods of time after this.

Optic nerve function should be monitored every 4 hours while the orbital cellulitis is in its acute phase. Pupil reactions, visual acuity, colour vision and brightness appreciation should form part of this monitoring, and the patient must have sufficient information and awareness of the condition to recognise the importance of these investigations at a time when he or she may well be feeling very ill.

Monitoring may be more of a problem in children with orbital cellulitis because it is likely that they will be in a specialist paediatric area where, although the nursing staff have a wealth of knowledge about the care of the sick child, they may know little about ophthalmic care and be unaware both of the tests that should take place and of their importance and significance. Ophthalmic clinicians must therefore be very clear in their handover of a child to a paediatric setting and may have to take responsibility for the ophthalmic care of the child through regular enquiries about the child's progress in the paediatric setting and by physically attending to ensure that investigations are carried out.

Surgery may be required to drain subperiosteal or orbital abscesses but medical management is sufficient in many cases (Garcia and Harris 2000).

Surgical drainage of an orbital abscess is indicated if any of the following occurs:

- A decrease in vision
- A relative afferent pupillary defect (RAPD) develops
- Proptosis progresses
- The size of the abscess does not reduce on CT within 48–72 hours of appropriate antibiotic administration. If brain abscesses develop and do not respond to antibiotic therapy, craniotomy is indicated (Harrington 2006).

Complications may be orbital or intracranial:

- Abscesses may occur in the orbit or sub-periorbitally.
- Corneal damage may occur as a result of exposure of neurotrophic keratitis.
- Ocular tissue may be damaged by secondary glaucoma, optic neuritis, central retinal artery occlusion (CRAO), or infection of the optic or oculomotor nerves or the extraocular muscles.
- Meningitis, cavernous sinus thrombosis and intercranial abscesses may occur and there is still a level of mortality associated with this condition.

REFERENCES

Ferguson MP, McNab AA (1999). Current treatment and outcome in orbital cellulitis. *Aust N Z J Ophthalmol* **27**:375–9.

Garcia GH, Harris GJ (2000). Criteria for nonsurgical management of subperiosteal abscess of the orbit: analysis of outcomes 1988–1998. *Ophthalmology* **107**:1454–6; discussion 1457–8.

Harrington J (2006). Orbital cellulites. Available at: www.emedicine. com/oph/topic205.htm (accessed 7 June 2007).

Rutar T, Zwick OM, Cockerham KP, Horton JC (2005). Bilateral blindness from orbital cellulitis caused by community-acquired methicillin-resistant *Staphylococcus aureus*. *Am J Ophthalmol* **140**: 740–2.

Chalazion (meibomian cysts)

4

4

DEFINITION

A chalazion is chronic inflammation of a meibomian gland (deep type) or zeisian sebaceous gland (superficial type), resulting in a clinically firm, painless nodule of the eyelid. Histologically, there is deep dermal or subcutaneous, suppurative, granulomatous inflammation containing neutrophils, plasma cells, lymphocytes, histiocytes and giant cells in a zonal configuration around central lipid material (Tasman and Jaeger 2002).

RISKS

Risks fall into two main areas: those of misdiagnosis and those of treatment options. Misdiagnosis includes missing those of other potential malignancy: sebaceous cell carcinoma, squamous cell carcinoma and basal cell carcinoma (BCC).

Risks in treatments include those related to incision and curettage, including incision of the lid line, incomplete removal of contents, infection, swelling and bruising.

SIGNS AND SYMPTOMS

The upper eyelids contain approximately 25 meibomian glands in each lid and approximately 20 in each lower lid. The patient gives a history of no trauma. A singular or multiple, firm, red nodule develops in the lid. This is variable in size and over some days can fluctuate in size. Depending on the location the patient will complain of varying degrees of irritation and watering. Chalazia in the central third of the upper lid can cause a mechanical astigmatism because the chalazion distorts the cornea on blinking. The nodule is mobile, often tender to touch (depending on size and tension). On occasion the cyst may rupture on either the

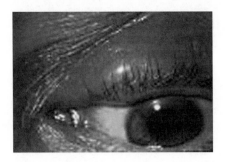

Figure 4.1 Chalazion.

conjunctival side or the skin side. If the cyst does rupture on the skin side, the wound may take several weeks to heal completely.

DIAGNOSIS
Diagnosis is by history and examination. Careful consideration of alternative diagnoses must be kept in mind.

CAUSES
There is a local reaction within the meibomian gland, which provokes an inflammatory response and results in the formation of a cyst. The contents of such cysts can be fluid or cheesy in consistency. Colour varies from clear to dark-green/brown. Clinically there appears to be a link between blepharitis and chalazion formation. The cyst may become infected, in which case the lid becomes swollen and red locally, and the area becomes very tender.

TREATMENT
The vast majority of chalazia will resolve spontaneously with no specific measures. Patients seem to find hot compresses and massage comforting and there are various rationales for this in texts (such as the heat may help antibiotics to absorb and help to liquefy secretions, and massage may help the chalazion to discharge). Various recommendations can be found in various texts

with little to support these claims other than practitioner evidence. In the absence of empirical evidence, however, massage and heat may help in individual patients, determined by a clinician's experience.

Infected chalazia require antibiotic therapy to deal with the infection and prevent extension of local infection to a wider area. Topical antibiotic ointment appears to be more effective, in general, than systemic antibiotics alone. Chalazia usually reduce to small, granulomatous lumps in the lid, which often resolve over a period of time. Unresolved chalazia may be felt to be cosmetically unacceptable or may cause continuing irritation. Cysts in the upper lid may cause a reversible astigmatic change that gets worse throughout the day because the chalazion is continually rubbed over the cornea as a result of lid movement (Kanski 2003). This tends to disappear overnight as the lid is closed. Often, further treatment of the chalazion is required.

Incision and curettage is a common minor operation to reduce chalazia. Under local anaesthetic (xylocaine 2%) and topical anaesthetic (such as oxybuprocaine 0.4%) the cyst is drained from a single tarsal incision, which allows the lid to act as its own bandage. Curettage removes the contents of the cyst and any redundant granulomatous tissue and, if the chalazion is recurrent, samples of tissue should be sent for histology. Topical antibiotics are required to prevent wound infection. Padding helps to stop bleeding and prevent bruising (McQueen 2006). An alternative version of the single incision is the American version where the cyst is incised parallel to the meibomian gland (as in the UK) and then perpendicular to the first incision. The centre of the incisions (the internal corners) is then lifted and removed with scissors to leave a space in the tarsal plate to drain secretions.

Triamcinolone (steroid) injections are gaining credibility in reducing chalazia and are popular in the USA. Side effects are for any steroid but lid skin discoloration is one that is specific to chalazion management. Khurana et al. (1988) demonstrated that steroid injection worked as well as surgery in some chalazia, but surgery was more effective for large lesions. Dhaliwal and Bhatia (2005) found that, where there is a purulent collection within the chalazion, surgery should also be the treatment of choice in patients aged over 35 years and for lesions with a duration of more than 8 months or a size > 11.4 mm. They found that smaller, harder lesions may be treated by either modality.

LIKELY PROGNOSIS
Prognosis is excellent. Occasionally cysts may recur; if they recur at the same site consider sebaceous cell carcinoma. Histological samples are recommended.

FOLLOW-UP CARE
None necessary. Advice should be given on seeking help if cysts persist or return.

PATIENT EDUCATION
Avoid the use of eye make-up during episodes of chalazion.

Hot compresses and massage techniques should be demonstrated to the patient.

Simple eye ointment, available from pharmacists, could help to provide symptomatic relief of ocular irritation.

REFERENCES
Dhaliwal U, Bhatia A (2005). A rationale for therapeutic decision making in chalazia. *Orbit* **24**:227–30.

Kanski JJ (2003). *Clinical Ophthalmology*, 5th edn. London: Butterworth-Heinemann.

Khurana AK, Ahluwalia BK, Rajan C (1988). Chalazion therapy. Intralesional steroids versus incision and curettage. *Acta Ophthalmol* **66**:352–4.

McQueen l (2006). Eyelids and lacrimal drainage system. In: Marsden J (ed.), *Ophthalmic Care*. Chichester: Wiley, 276–306.

Tasman W, Jaeger E (2002). *Duane's Clinical Ophthalmology*. New York: Lippincott, Williams & Wilkins.

Dry eye syndrome

5

'Dry eye' is a general term used to describe a disease resulting from inadequate wetting of the cornea and conjunctiva by the precorneal tear film (PCTF). Millions of people worldwide suffer from dry eye.

Despite its high prevalence, dry eye is not always easy to diagnose. The vast majority of patients have symptoms that are mild to moderate in severity. Although these patients have genuine discomfort, objective signs of dry eye may be missed and, without proper diagnosis, patients may not receive the attention and treatment that this condition warrants.

SIGNS AND SYMPTOMS

The signs and symptoms of dry eye can be misinterpreted as evidence of other conditions such as infectious, allergic or irritative conjunctivitis.

The symptoms vary considerably from one individual to another. Most patients complain of a foreign body sensation, burning and general ocular discomfort. The discomfort is typically described as scratchy, dry, sore, gritty, smarting or burning. Discomfort is the hallmark of dry eye because the cornea is richly supplied with sensory nerve fibres.

A significant percentage of patients also experience photophobia and intermittent blurring or other problems with visual acuity.

Individuals with dry eye commonly remark that their eyes tire easily, making it difficult for them to read or watch television. The reason for this difficulty is that the frequency of blinking typically decreases during tasks that require concentration. As blink frequency decreases, there is more time for the tear film to evaporate. If blinking is sufficiently infrequent, the duration of exposure will exceed the tear film break-up time (BUT), resulting in the formation of one or more dry spots on the corneal surface (Lamberts 2005).

Contact lens intolerance can also be a symptom of dry eye. Sometimes, a patient with mild-to-moderate dry eye may not experience symptoms until contact lenses are fitted, the placement of which can upset the delicate balance of tear film production and distribution, leading to lens intolerance.

CAUSES

Dry eye may be caused by immunological conditions such as rheumatoid arthritis, Sjögren syndrome, systemic lupus erythematosus (SLE) or inflammatory damage to the tear gland. Generally it is associated with age and called 'keratoconjunctivitis sicca'. Current theory suggests that dry eye syndrome results from lymphocytes infiltrating the lacrimal gland and causing chronic progressive inflammation (Stern et al. 1998). It is also suggested that levels of androgens that protect the ocular surface from inflammation decrease with age and, when the level is reduced (as at the menopause), ocular cells make more cytokines that attract T cells to the conjunctiva, producing surface damage and increasing symptoms of dry eye.

Dry eye conditions are classified as various types of abnormalities that can lead to insufficient wetting of the cornea.

CLASSIFICATION
- Abnormalities of the aqueous layer
- Abnormalities of the mucin layer
- Abnormalities of the lipid layer
- Abnormalities of the corneal epithelium
- Abnormalities of the lids.

Abnormalities of the aqueous layer
Insufficient production of the aqueous component of the tear film is the most common cause of dry eye. The resulting condition, known as keratoconjunctivitis sicca (KCS), is usually the result of decreased tear production by the accessory lacrimal glands. Inflammation of the lacrimal glands may be accompanied by

inflammation and drying of other mucous membranes, particularly those in the mouth, vagina and/or respiratory tract.

Abnormalities of the mucin layer

Deficient production of mucin interferes with the even distribution (spreading) of the tear film across the corneal surface, resulting in a very unstable and uneven tear film with a rapid BUT. Abnormalities in the mucin layer of the PCTF often occur as a result of loss of the goblet cells of the conjunctival epithelium.

Abnormalities of the lipid layer

When abnormalities in the lipid layer of the PCTF occur, deficiencies in the lipid layer result in excessive evaporation of the aqueous component of the tear film, which in turn leads to drying of the ocular surface.

Abnormalities of the corneal epithelium

Alterations in the normal morphology of the corneal epithelium, which can adversely affect tear film stability, are called epithelial cell defects. Infections and trauma resulting in corneal scars and ulcerations can damage the microvilli, causing permanent dry spots. Damage to the corneal surface can also result from exposure to certain drugs, including many types of general anaesthetics.

Abnormalities of the lids

As the eyelids play such an important role in distributing the tear film, normal blinking is essential to maintaining healthy corneal and conjunctival surfaces. Thus, anything that interferes with normal blinking, or anatomical abnormalities that interfere with complete closure of the eyelids during blinking, can result in drying of the ocular surface.

TREATMENT

The nature of this disease can be complex but the mainstay choice of therapy is often determined based on the severity of symptoms (Brewitt and Sistani 2001). The most widely used therapy is tear replacement by topical artificial tears. The goal is to increase humidity at the ocular surface, to improve lubrication and thus decrease symptoms (Calonge 2001).

An increasing body of evidence is demonstrating that the use of ciclosporin reverses inflammation on the ocular surface and thus alleviates patients' symptoms (Turner et al. 2000). By decreasing inflammation, and augmenting the oil and water layers of the tear film, omega 3 supplementation looks promising as an oral treatment (Boerner 2000), but further studies are required for full evaluation of the magnitude of its efficacy in treating patients with dry eye. Autologous serum tears have been used in severe dry eye to good effect (Rocha et al. 2000); these bypass the problems associated with preservatives in long-term drop use.

In general the following is a quick guide to current evidence-based treatments, but finding a regimen that suits the individual is usually by trial and error:

- Mild cases of dry eye, in which there are no signs of significant damage to the cornea or conjunctiva, can usually be managed with artificial tears.
- Moderate cases need artificial tears and possibly lubricating ointments at night.
- In addition to the above, severe cases characterised by keratinisation of the conjunctiva, which may include punctate keratopathy and filaments, and may require acetylcysteine 5% (Dentinger et al. 2000), anti-inflammatory preparations and additional tear-preserving therapies such as punctal occlusion to prevent loss of natural tears.
- Patients with posterior marginal blepharitis (meibomian gland dysfunction) will need a lid hygiene regimen of warm compresses followed by lid scrubs (Shaw 2002; Chew et al. 2003), as well as topical antibiotics. Tetracycline or the derivate doxycycline is currently the treatment of choice (Torbit and Sutton 1996).

EXPECTATIONS (PROGNOSIS)
Most patients with dry eye have only discomfort, and no vision loss. With severe cases, the cornea may become damaged or infected.

COMPLICATIONS
Ulcers or infections of the cornea are serious complications.

GENERAL TREATMENT GUIDELINES FOR NURSES FOR
FIRST-LINE THERAPY
One of the most important drawbacks is that many artificial tears
contain preservatives, the most common of which is benzalko-
nium chloride (BAK). The prolonged presence of artificial tears
on an already compromised ocular surface can worsen the disease
and thus the symptoms (Burstein 1980; Lopez Bernal and Ubels
1991). If signs of allergic reaction appear switch to preservative-
free drops.

If underlying pathology is detected, where possible treatment
should be directed towards caustive factor (that is, lid hygiene
and antibiotics for blepharitis).

Start with a polyvinylalcohol (PVA) preparation
- PVA 1% (Hypo Tears) – preservative BAK
- PVA 1.4% (Sno Tears) – preservative chlorobutanol.

Rationale: these mucomimetics are cheap, do not cause crusting
or blurring and may offer symptomatic relief. However, they
have a poor retention time.

If symptoms and discomfort persist
In this case consider a polyacrylic acid gel (PAA).

- PAA 0.2% (Viscotears) – preservative cetrimide 0.1 mg/g.

Rationale: longer retention time may therefore improve patient
compliance and can be given twice daily. It can stabilise the tear
film for up to 6 h (Bron et al. 1998). Cetrimide preservative is not
as toxic as BAK.

Other products
Other products that may be of use as an adjunctive to the above,
depending on pathology of deficient tear film, are:

- Lubricant ointment (Lacri-Lube) – preservative
  chlorobutanol.

Rationale: effective in preventing tear evaporation. Only small amount needed to give corneal protection. Best used at night because it is very viscous and blurs vision.

- Punctal occlusion: surgical for permanent or plugging for temporary or semi-temporary occlusion.

Rationale: for moderate-to-severe dry eyes in order to prevent drainage of tears, thus conserve natural tears or retain artificial ones. Consider only when dry eye is not controlled by other methods (Committee on Ophthalmic Procedure Assessment 1997; Yen et al. 2001).

Preservative-free tear subsitutes are also available – Minims artificial tears and Celluvisc are common.

HEALTH EDUCATION

It is important that the patients get the time, support and education that they require to understand and live with the condition. General advice should include the following:

- Instillation and compliance with treatment therapy: in general, the only person who can control the symptoms is the patient and he or she must be encouraged to find a regimen that works – using drops before the eye becomes irritated. Ophthalmic health-care professionals can advise, but are not a substitute for a patient who is an expert in the condition.
- Possibility of discontinuing contact lenses use, reducing wear time – or using frequent, unpreserved drops.
- Avoidance or reduction in activities that reduce blinking, for example, reading, driving, working on a computer monitor or watching television – or at least, being aware that these activities will aggravate the condition, so that patients can use tear substitutes more frequently.
- Reducing exposure to fumes, dust, cigarette smoke and dry air-conditioned or centrally heated environments, which can aggravate symptoms – a bowl of water placed in the room may help to raise humidity levels and decrease symptoms.

REFERENCES

Boerner CF (2000). Dry eye successfully treated with oral flaxseed oil. *Ocular Surgery News* **15**:147–8.

Brewitt H, Sistani F (2001). Dry eye disease: The scale of the problem. *Surv Ophthalmol* **45**(suppl 2):S199–201.

Bron A, Mangat H, Quinlan M (1998). Polyacrylic acid gel in patients with dry eyes: a randomised comparison with polyvinylalcohol. *Eur J Ophthalmol* **8**:81–9.

Burstein NL (1980). Corneal cytotoxicity of topically applied drugs, vehicles and preservatives. *Surv Ophthalmol* **25**:15–30.

Calonge M (2001). The treatment of dry eye. *Surv Ophthalmol* **45**(suppl 2):S227–39.

Chew C, James B, Bron A (2003). *Ophthalmology*, 9th edn. Oxford: Blackwell.

Committee on Ophthalmic Procedure Assessment (1997). Punctal occlusion for the dry eye. *Ophthalmology* **104**:1521–4.

Dentinger PJ, Swenson CF, Anaizi NH (2000). Stability of famotidine in extemporaneously compounded oral liquid. *Am J Syst Pharm* **57**:1340–2.

Lamberts DW (2005). Dry eyes. In: *The Cornea: Scientific foundation and clinical practice*, 4th edn. Philadelphia: Lippincott, William & Wilkins.

Lopez Bernal D, Ubels JL (1991). Quantitative evaluation of the corneal epithelial barrier: effect of artificial tears and preservatives. *Curr Eye Res* **10**:645–56.

Rocha EM, Pelegrino FSA, de Paiv CS, Vigorito AC, de Souza CA (2000). GVHD dry eyes treated with autologous serum tears. *Bone Marrow Transplant* **25**:1101–3.

Shaw M (2002). Recognising and managing blepharitis. *Ophthal Nursing* **6**(2):22–5.

Stern ME, Beuerman RW, Fox RI et al. (1998). The pathology of dry eye; the interaction between the ocular surface and lacrimal gland. *Cornea* **17**:584–9.

Torbit JK, Sutton BM (1996). Clinical practice guidelines: Ocular surface disease. *Clinical Eye Care Vision Care* **8**:197–201.

Turner K, Pflugfelder SC, Ji Z (2000). Interleukin-6 levels in the conjunctival epithelium of patients with dry eye disease treated with cyclosporine ophthalmic emulsion. *Cornea* **19**:492–6.

Yen MT, Pflugfelder SC, Feuer WJ (2001). The effect of punctal occlusion on tear production, tear clearance, and ocular surface sensation in normal subjects. *Am J Ophthalmol* **131**:314–23.

5

Ectropion

DEFINITION

An ectropion is malposition of the lower eyelid in an outward and/or droopy position. It can be congenital or acquired. Acquired ectropion may be classified as involutional, mechanical, cicatricial or paralytic (Beaconsfield 2001).

RISKS

The risks of ectropion range from abnormal watering of the eye as a result of malposition of the puncta and the lid margin, to conjunctival and corneal damage.

SIGNS AND SYMPTOMS

Patients in the early stages complain of disturbed vision as a result of abnormal tearing, which may be associated with irritation of the cornea. Some patients complain of recurring infection of the eye (Fraser et al. 2001). Symptoms may be worsened by winter-like weather, particularly windy cold days. As the ectropion worsens the lid droops away from the globe, making the patient's symptoms constant and more severe. Cosmetically the patient has varying amounts of the lower fornix exposed, which can cause social embarrassment.

DIAGNOSIS

Diagnosis is confirmed by careful ophthalmic history taking and examination of the lids, taking careful note of the position of the lids in relation to the globes. Where there is evidence of epiphora and lid malposition, ectropion can be suspected.

CAUSES

Congenital ectropion is probably caused by spasm of orbicularis oculi and is more common in children with Down syndrome because of skin shortening. Mechanical ectropion is caused by lid lesions. Involutional ectropion is caused by laxity of the lower lid skin and usually involves the lower puncta. When it does involve the puncta, the patient invariably complains of severe tearing. Cicatricial ectropion is caused by scarring of the surrounding tissues, commonly in ocular pemphigoid. Paralytic ectropion is usually caused by a facial nerve palsy (McQueen 2006).

TREATMENTS

Treatment is geared towards symptomatic relief of the underlying causes. Initial treatment is usually lubricants for the conjunctiva/cornea when irritation becomes a problem.

- Mechanical ectropion is commonly managed by surgical correction of the manifesting lid pathology.
- Involutional ectropion is usually surgically managed and may involve lid shortening.
- Cicatricial ectropion is treated by removal of the scar tissue or abnormal skin using Z-plasty.
- Paralytic ectropion is treated with copious lubricants to prevent corneal damage; in some cases it may require lateral tarsorrhaphy.

LIKELY PROGNOSIS

The prognosis is good. Patients can be impatient with non-surgical management; prompt education is important to gain compliance and concordance with the agreed management plan. Surgical intervention should consist of the minimum surgery required to resolve the problem.

Ectropion can recur after surgical correction as the skin and underlying structures become lax during the ageing process.

FOLLOW-UP CARE

Patients will need to be monitored regularly to assess state of regression or egression of the ectropion. Patients who have had corrective surgery can be discharged from immediate care once the wound has healed.

PATIENT EDUCATION

Comprehensive information should be provided to the patient verbally and in written format. Non-surgical management can at first be complicated for new patients and it is important that the health-care practitioner ensures that the patient understands the importance of the management and the problems that can occur if treatment is not adhered to.

REFERENCES

Beaconsfield M (2001). Ectropion. In: Collin R, Rose G (eds), *Plastic and Orbital Surgery*. London: BMJ Books, 15–23.

Fraser S, Asaria R, Kon C (2001). *Eye Know How*. London: BMJ Books.

McQueen L (2006). Eyelids and lacrimal drainage system. In: Marsden J (ed.), *Ophthalmic Care*. Chichester: Wiley, 276–306.

6

Entropion

7

DEFINITION

An entropion is malposition of the lower eyelid in an inward position. Three types have been identified: involutional or age related, cicatricial and congenital (Beaconsfield 2001).

RISKS

The risk in entropion is to the cornea. The malposition of the lower lid (being turned in) causes corneal irritation and, in some cases, corneal damage. Compromised corneas can lead to keratitis caused by opportunistic organisms. Entropion may cause the patient irritation and discomfort, but a longstanding entropion can lead to severe corneal desiccation.

SIGNS AND SYMPTOMS

Patients usually complain of the vision being altered by too many tears as a result of corneal irritation increasing the blink rate. The lower lid may not visibly show any signs of 'turning in' on gross inspection, with the patient's symptoms seemingly being more intermittent or severe than the clinical findings suggest. Latterly the patient may present with foreign body sensation, watering and red eye.

DIAGNOSIS

Diagnosis is by careful ophthalmic history taking of the complaint. Symptoms are usually expressed by the patient as slowly getting worse with incremental severity of symptoms. The irregularity of the symptoms has gradually become constant. Examination of the lids may show both lashes and lid margin turning inwards. Looking at the palpebral conjunctiva may show fibrosed shallow recesses, particularly if caused by ocular pemphigoid.

Lax retractors (and therefore entropion) can be identified in most cases by asking the patient to squeeze the eyelids tightly shut a few times and observing the resultant lid position. This action obliges the orbicularis to turn the lid inwards if the retractors are lax.

CAUSES

Involutional entropion is caused by the lower lid retractors becoming lax, enabling the lid to move out of position laterally. The preseptal orbicularis action overrides the pretarsal orbicularis and tips the lid inwards (Kanski 2003).

Cicatricial entropion caused by scarring on the conjunctiva in the fornices pulls the lid inward.

Congenital entropion is said to be rare and mostly encountered among people of Oriental racial origin.

TREATMENTS

Some laxity in the early stages can be reclaimed with regular skin massage over the area of the entropion. Moisturising creams such as E45 assist in the reversal of laxity, but this is a first aid measure and cannot prevent the advancement of the entropion long term. Besides symptomatic help, such as epilation of lashes temporarily in the wrong position as a result of lid malposition, taping the lid to evert it slightly and lubricants, the only permanent solution is surgery. Such procedures as Weiss sutures and Quickert's procedure realign the lids to a more normal position.

LIKELY PROGNOSIS

The prognosis is excellent. Difficulties that arise early are patients' willingness to accept partnership in helping themselves to reduce the laxity with regular massage. Ignoring the immediate post-operative care, post-surgery, patients may experience some weeks of pain, which they should be advised of before the surgery. Overcorrection of the laxity can lead to a set of problems that are best avoided, such as tearing, pain and asymmetry of lid position. Patients having corrective entropion surgery should be advised that the laxity might return in years to come.

FOLLOW-UP CARE

There is no specific follow-up care with successful surgical correction.

PATIENT EDUCATION

Patients yet to undergo surgical correction should have lid massage demonstrated to them and be encouraged to adopt massage as part of their daily routine.

REFERENCES

Beaconsfield M (2001). Ectropion. In: Collin R, Rose G (eds), *Plastic and Orbital Surgery*. London: BMJ Books, 15–23.

Kanski J (2003). *Clinical Ophthalmology*, 5th edn. London: Butterworth-Heinemann.

7

Infestation of lashes: phthiriasis palpebrum

The louse – *Phthirus pubis* – is adapted to live in pubic hair but may be transmitted to other hair-covered areas, particularly the eyelashes. It is the only louse likely to be found in this area. Lice on lashes cause irritation and itching and are often found in children. Although sexual abuse should be considered, transmission from vectors such as pillows and sheets is most likely, as well as indirect contact from infested carers (Lopez Garcia et al. 2003). The lice must not merely be pulled from lashes, because they tend to bury their heads in the skin of the lid, and body parts such as the head or legs may be left behind. Kanski (2003) suggests trimming lashes at their base or the use of mercuric oxide 1% ointment (not available in the UK). He also recommends anticholinesterase agents, laser or cryotherapy as treatment options. Lopez Garcia et al. (2003) consider these treatments and others, many of which are very toxic to the eye (for example, chemicals in alcohol), do not kill the louse eggs (for example, fluorescein 20%) or would not be possible in children (for example, lash cutting, laser or cryotherapy). They recommend malathion, an anticholinesterase, in a water rather than an alcohol base, applied to the lid margin in a single application by a health professional, and left unwashed for 24 hours, to kill both lice and eggs. The *British National Formulary* (BMA, RPSGB 2007) also suggests aqueous malathion (for example, Derbac M) for lice on eyelashes.

The treatment of phthiriasis palpebrum is therefore malathion, in aqueous solution, applied to the lid margin in a single application by a health professional, and left unwashed for 24 hours.

REFERENCES

British Medical Association, Royal Pharmaceutical Society of Great Britain (2007). *British National Formulary 54*. London: BMA/RPSGB.

Kanski JJ (2003). *Clinical Ophthalmology*, 5th edn. London: Butterworth-Heinemann.

Lopez Garcia JS, Garcia Lozano I, Matrinez Garclintonena J (2003). Phthiriasis palpebrum: diagnosis and treatment. *Archiv Sociedad Española Oftalmol* **78**:365–74.

Lid eversion

9

Upper lid eversion is often required to search for conjunctival foreign bodies or other conjunctival signs. The patient is asked to look down and the examiner grasps the eyelashes of the upper lid between the thumb and the index finger, with the finger on top (Figure 9.1). A cotton-tipped applicator – held like a pencil and pointing downwards – is used to press gently (but firmly) downwards over the superior aspect of the tarsal plate (Figure 9.2). The tarsal plate will be felt to evert and the edge of the lid can be moved slightly backwards and kept in place by the thumb on the lashes (Figure 9.3 and 9.4). The patient should continue to look down to expose as much of the tarsal conjunctiva as possible. The examiner should have a penlight within reach to inspect the exposed conjunctival surface of the upper lid for a foreign body or other abnormality. Any foreign body may be wiped off with the cotton-tipped applicator. To return the lid to its normal position, the examiner releases the lid margin and the patient is instructed to look up.

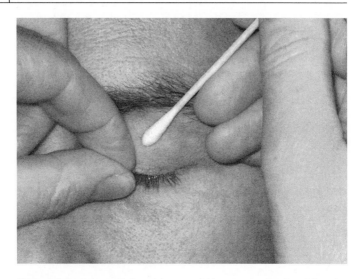

Figure 9.1 Grasp the eye lashes of the upper lid between the thumb and the index finger, with the finger on top.

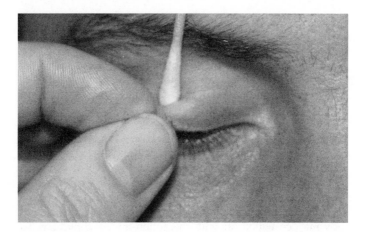

Figure 9.2 Press gently, but firmly downwards over the superior aspect of the tarsal plate.

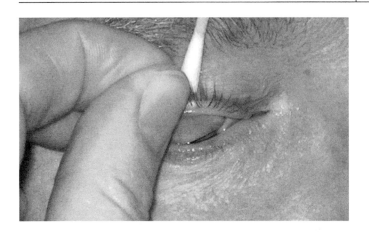

Figure 9.3 The tarsal plate will evert and the edge of the lid can be moved slightly backwards.

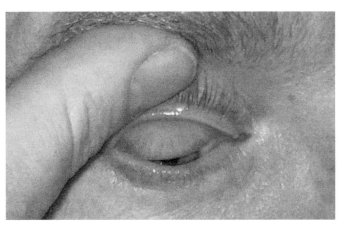

Figure 9.4 Keep the lid in place with the thumb on the lashes.

Attempts should not be made to 'wrap' the lid around the cotton-tipped applicator or manipulate the lid to evert. It will evert well with minimum pressure in the correct place and this option is much less uncomfortable for the patient.

Sac wash-out (irrigation of the lacrimal ducts)

This procedure is carried out to assess the patency of the nasolacrimal system in patients with excessive tearing.

Tears drain via the upper and lower puncta and canaliculi into the lacrimal sac. The nasolacrimal duct proceeds down to the inferior meatus of the nasal cavity.

There are a number of causes for defective drainage of tears through the lacrimal passages:

- Facial palsy: weakness of orbicularis oculi, which impairs the pumping action of the canaliculi
- Punctal malposition: ectropion and entropion
- Punctal occlusion: congenital absence, scarring, blockage as a result, for example, of chronic infection with staphylococci, Streptothrix sp. or herpes simplex, or after long-term drug administration
- Canalicular obstruction secondary to canaliculitis.

Many elderly patients get stenosis of the nasolacrimal duct, which leads to epiphora and a mucopurulent discharge (Haeringhen 1997). Secondary infection is common, producing an acute dacryocystitis with abscess formation. The swelling is frequently painful. Stenosis may be bypassed by dacryocystorhinostomy (DCR). Alternatives to surgical DCR include endonasal laser DCR and nasolacrimal duct balloon dilatation or stenting. Acute dacryocystitis may be treated with systemic antibiotics.

A simple fluorescein dye disappearance test may be helpful to assess the patency of the lacrimal system – a small drop of fluorescein 2% is instilled into both eyes. This will normally disappear over 5 min if the duct is patent, and may subsequently be visible in the nostril using blue light or on a tissue if you ask the patient to blow his or her nose.

In infants, the problem can be caused by incomplete canalisation of the lower end of the duct. The nasolacrimal duct does not cannulate until birth, and there may be a persistent membranous obstruction at the bottom end of the nasolacrimal duct in up to 70% of neonates (dacryostenosis). Spontaneous resolution occurs in most cases – 20% of babies will still have symptoms at age 1 month, with less than 1% still having symptoms at age 1 year (Young and MacEwen 1997). Most cases resolve spontaneously within 10 months of birth. Antibiotic eye ointment is indicated if there is infection but, if it persists, patency of the nasolacrimal duct may be explored by syringing (Paul and Shepherd 1994).

CLINICAL PRACTICE

Observe a clean dressing technique throughout.

Equipment: Nettleship dilator, lacrimal cannula, 2 mL syringe, ampoule or sachet of sodium chloride 0.9%, 21 mm hypodermic needle, dressing pack.

The procedure is not painful but may be a little uncomfortable. A topical anaesthetic drop is often instilled before the procedure but it has little effect in anaesthetising the canalicular pathways (McQueen 2006).

- Explain the procedure to the patient and position him or her in a chair with the head supported to prevent movement during the procedure.
- Instil a drop of local anaesthetic directly on to the punctum to achieve optimum comfort for the patient.
- Draw up sodium chloride into the 2 mL syringe, attach the lacrimal cannula and check patency by expressing a small amount through the lumen.
- Ask the patient to look up temporally when syringing the lower punctum and down and laterally if you wish to syringe the upper punctum. This protects the cornea from any accidental abrasion.
- Using the Nettleship dilator, insert the point approximately 2 mm into the punctum and gently rotate for a few seconds in a nasal direction to relax and dilate the punctum, before removing it very gently. This is useful if punctal stenosis is present;

10

however, if the bore of the lacrimal cannula is smaller than the punctum, it is not necessary.

- Introduce the lacrimal cannula, into the lower punctum first, in a downward and then horizontal direction, following the pathway of the canaliculus. The cannula should be pushed, very gently until a 'stop' is felt (the medial wall of the lacrimal sac and lacrimal bone). Ease the cannula back gently away from this and then inject the sodium chloride slowly while observing for any regurgitation through either punctum.
- Ask the patient if he or she has tasted or felt anything in the back of the throat that would indicate patency of the system.
- Partial obstruction in the canaliculus may be felt as a slight resistance on insertion and partial obstruction; lower in the lacrimal system resistance may be felt when injecting and a delay may be experienced before saline is felt by the patient in the throat.
- Complete obstruction of the canaliculus will be felt as a 'soft stop' rather than the 'hard stop' at the lacrimal sac. Obstruction below the common canaliculus will result in regurgitation through the upper punctum. No saline will travel as far as the throat.
- Repeat on other puncta as requested and document findings in the patient's notes.
- The more skilled the clinician becomes, the more descriptive and useful the findings of the procedure can be and these can inform treatment options.

REFERENCES

Haeringhen N (1997). Aging and the lacrimal system. *Br J Ophthalmol* **81**:824–6.

McQueen L (2006). Eyelids and lacrimal drainage system. In: Marsden J (ed.), *Ophthalmic Care*. Chichester: Wiley, 276–306.

Paul T, Shepherd R (1994). Congenital nasolacrimal duct obstruction: natural history and the timing of optimal intervention. *J Pediatr Ophthalmol Strabismus* **31**:362–7.

Young JD, MacEwen CJ (1997). Managing congenital lacrimal obstruction in general practice. *BMJ* **315**:293–6.

10

Schirmer's tear test

DEFINITION

Schirmer's tear test is a simple and inexpensive way of determining tear production for a given individual at the time of testing. The test is commonly used if a patient is experiencing symptoms associated with dry eye or has excessive watering of the eyes, to exclude or help diagnose keratoconjunctivitis sicca. The test measures basic tear function. Even though it has been available for over a century, several clinical studies have shown that it does not properly identify a large group of patients with dry eyes as a result of its crude methodology and user variability (Alfonso et al. 1999).

One test that is not commonly used, but is scientifically more accurate and, therefore worth noting, is lacrimal scintigraphy (Gencoglue et al. 2005). This is a non-invasive, practical, safe, simple imaging technique using a special camera that gives a quantitative assessment of the rate of drainage and measurement of tear clearance.

Another test used in the USA involving fluorescein also claims that it accurately measures the flow of dye out of the eye. It involves the use of a diagnostic kit containing a unit-dose dropper with 2–5 mL 2% fluorescein and a colour standard plate that is used to grade the concentration of fluorescein visually in the tear fluid 15 min after instillation of the dye (Pflugfelder et al. 2000).

METHOD FOR PERFORMING SCHIRMER'S TEAR TEST

Both eyes are tested at the same time. It is best to carry out the test in a dimly lit room to prevent tearing as a result of photophobia (Prabhasawat and Tseng 1998). If the patient is wearing contact lenses these should be removed 24 hours before the test if possible (Gencoglue et al. 2005). A standard Schirmer strip of

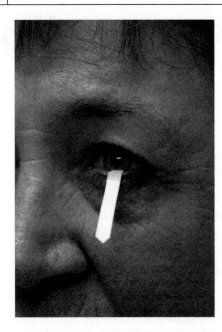

Figure 11.1 Schirmer's tear test. Reproduced with permission of the Ophthalmic Imaging Department, Flinders Medical Centre, South Australia.

filter paper is placed inside in the inferolateral third of the lower eyelid, taking care to prevent contact of the paper with the cornea. The patient is asked to close the eyes or look in an upward gaze for 5 min. After this time, the paper is removed and the amount of wetting on the strip measured (in millimetres).

The types of Schirmer's tear test are described by Smith et al. (2004) and in *The Eye Digest* (www.agingeye.net/dryeyes/dryeyeseyeexam.php):

- Schirmer 1: without anaesthetic which measures basal + reflex secretion
- Schirmer 2: with anaesthetic, which measures basal tear secretion
- Schirmer 3: when the nasal mucosa is irritated with a cotton-tipped applicator to provoke further reflex tearing.

11

CONSIDERATIONS
- If the patient cannot tolerate the tear strip without topical anaesthetic, the test should be recorded as done with anaesthetic, or Schirmer 2.
- The test should be performed before any topical medication or manipulation of the eyelid.
- If the patient wishes to close the eyes during the test he or she should be informed to do this gently. Tight closing of the eyes or rubbing them during the test can cause abnormal test results as a result of stimulation of tears or result in a superficial corneal abrasion (from the test strip).

INTERPRETATION OF RESULTS
More than 10 mm of moisture on the strip is normal. Below 5 mm in 5 min is abnormal and warrants further investigation.

REFERENCES

Alfonso A, Monroy D, Stern ME, Feuer WJ, Tseng SCG, Pflugfelder SC (1999). Correlation of tear fluorescein clearance and Schirmer test scores with ocular irritation symptoms. *Ophthalmology* **106**: 803–10.

Gencoglue EA, Dursun D, Akova YA, Cengiz F (2005). Tear clearance measurement in patients with dry eye syndrome using quantitative lacrimal scintigraphy. *Ann Nuclear Med* **19**:581–7.

Pflugfelder SC, Solomon A, Stern ME (2000). The diagnosis and management of dry eye: a twenty-five-year review. *Cornea* **9**:644–9.

Prabhasawat P, Tseng SCG (1998). Frequent association of delayed tear clearance in ocular irritation. *Br J Ophthalmol* **82**:666–75.

Smith JA, Vitale S, Reed GF et al. (2004). Dry eye signs and symptoms in women with premature ovarian failure. *Arch Ophthalmol* **122**: 151–6.

The Tear film break-up time

The precorneal tear film is crucial to the maintenance of the optical health of the anterior surface of the eye. It acts as a vehicle for elimination of debris that accumulates, including endothelial cells, microbes and other waste. The tear film also helps regulate epithelial cell production, aiding repair and ongoing replacement of the epithelial layer (Lemp 2005).

Tears leave the surface of the eye through the puncta and the lacrimal drainage system, and by the process of evaporation.

Rapid tear film break-up time (BUT) is indicative of a deficit in the quality or quantity of one or more of the tear components. It can also be caused by an irregular anterior corneal surface, for example, superficial epithelial erosions. Fagien (1999) agrees that indicators of a deficiency in the qualitative component of the tear film may be best detected by assessing the tear film BUT.

Tears are spread over the anterior surface of the eye by the action of blinking. The tear film normally begins to thin after between 10 and 30 seconds; this causes dry spots, which are randomly distributed as they appear on the corneal surface.

The tear film BUT is measured as the time between the blink of the eyelid and the appearance of the first dry spot on the corneal surface. If the tear film is normal, the BUT is greater than the interval between blinks; this ensures that the integrity of the tear film remains constant, so continuously protecting the cornea.

The tear film BUT is measured using slit-lamp examination. A moistened strip or drop of fluorescein is applied into the lower fornix. After instillation, the patient is asked to blink several times and then not to blink until completion of the assessment. Observation of the cornea is carried out using a wide beam setting and cobalt blue filter light. The assessment is then timed. Tear

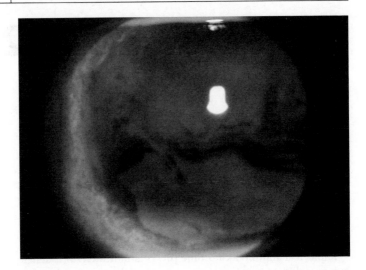

Figure 12.1 Tear film.

film BUT is noted when the first dark spot or lines are observed in the tear film, which is otherwise stained by the fluorescein dye (McQueen 2006). These dark areas are dry spots where the cornea is not protected by the tear film.

Tear film BUT < 10s is regarded as abnormal and a clinically significant sign of dry eye. It does not, however, identify the type of dry eye (Kanski 2003).

REFERENCES

Fagien S (1999). The value of tear film break-up and Schirmer's tests in preoperative blepharoplasty evaluation. *Plastic Reconstruct Surg* **104**:570–3.

Kanski J (2003). *Clinical Ophthalmology: A systematic approach*, 5th edn. London: Butterworth-Heinemann.

Lemp M (2005). Tear film evaluation. In: Krachmer J, Mannis M, Holland E (eds), *Cornea*, 2nd edn. London: Elsevier Mosby, 225–8.

McQueen L (2006). Eyelids and lacrimal drainage system. In: Marsden J (ed.), *Ophthalmic Care*. Chichester: Wiley, 276–306.

Section 2

Conjunctiva

Conjunctivitis

13

Conjunctivitis is a very common condition and accounts for many of the cases of 'red eye' presenting to primary and secondary care. Although often presumed to be mainly bacterial, the vast majority of cases of conjunctivitis in adults are viral in origin (Wishart et al. 1984; Tullo and Donnelly 1995). An accurate history and examination make differentiation between types of conjunctivitis fairly straightforward.

BACTERIAL CONJUNCTIVITIS

In acute bacterial conjunctivitis, the eyes become red and inflamed. The eyes are sticky throughout the day and profuse purulent discharge is evident, with the lashes often becoming stuck together. It is common in children, usually starting in one eye and spreading to the other, and its severity depends on the causative organism. The condition is not normally serious and usually recedes spontaneously within about a week. *Staphylococcus* spp. are the most common pathogens for bacterial conjunctivitis in adults, followed by *Streptococcus pneumoniae* and *Haemophilus influenzae* (Seal et al. 1982; Miller et al. 1992). In children, bacterial conjunctivitis is more common than the viral form and is mainly caused by *H. influenzae*, *S. pneumoniae* and *Moraxella catarrhalis* (Gigliotti et al. 1981; Weiss et al. 1993).

People with acute bacterial conjunctivitis are often given antibiotics, usually as eyedrops or ointment, to speed recovery. Use of antibiotics is associated with significantly improved rates of clinical and microbial remission, but the benefits are marginal because the condition resolves spontaneously in most cases. Sheikh and Hurwitz (2006) found a 65% cure or significant improvement rate with placebo in 2–5 days.

In children, Rose et al. (2005) suggest that most children with acute infective conjunctivitis in primary care will get better by themselves and do not need treatment with an antibiotic. Normann et al. (2002) found that chloramphenicol and fucithalmic were equally effective in treating neonates with bacterial conjunctivitis, but that fucithalmic was easier to use.

VIRAL CONJUNCTIVITIS
Viral conjunctivitis accounts for most adult conjunctivitis. In viral conjunctivitis, the eye is red and very irritable. Follicles are found under the upper lid, and often in the lower fornix and on the bulbar conjunctiva. The lids may be thickened as a result of general swelling. The eye is likely to be very watery, and sticky only in the morning as a result of dried tear secretions overnight. Viral conjunctivitis usually becomes bilateral. It may be associated with general malaise, a sore throat, and swollen submandibular and preauricular lymph nodes.

Adenovirus is the usual causative organism and different types may cause different clusters of symptoms. Type 13 causes pharyngoconjunctival fever (sore throat, conjunctivitis, generalised illness) and type 8 is known as epidemic keratoconjunctivitis (the cornea is severely affected).

Treatment is educative and supportive; the patient must be aware of the progress of the illness – it may take 2–3 weeks to settle and spread to the other eye, the patient may feel generally unwell and there is no effective treatment.

Artificial tears help to stabilise the tear film, which is disrupted as a result of continual lacrimation. They may be used very frequently for comfort. A dry eye may persist for some time after the infection has resolved.

CHLAMYDIAL CONJUNCTIVITIS
Chlamydial conjunctivitis typically affects sexually active young people, especially men and women aged under 25, and is the most frequent infectious cause of neonatal conjunctivitis in the USA. The US Centers for Disease Control (CDC) recognise *Chlamydia* sp. as one of the major sexually transmitted pathogens, estimating approximately three million new cases per year in the

USA (www.revoptom.com/handbook/SECT2D.HTM) and the picture is similar in scale in the UK with chlamydia infection being the most commonly diagnosed sexually transmitted infection (STI). Women seem to be more susceptible than men. Presentation is usually of a chronically red and irritable eye, which never progresses to the full-blown symptoms of viral or bacterial conjunctivitis, but just 'grumbles' along with no resolution. Large follicles are often found, especially in the lower fornix.

Chlamydia sp. should be suspected in a person with a unilateral, chronic conjunctivitis and swabs should be taken for chlamydia culture/PCR or polymerase chain reaction (often the swabs and culture medium are the same as those used for genital chlamydial culture). Sensitivity is important in dealing with this and the patient must give informed consent for the tests, as for every other intervention. Referral to a sexual health clinic is required, but only after a positive swab result has been received. It should be noted that most chlamydial infection goes undiagnosed (Department of Health 2007: www.dh.gov.uk/en/Policyandguidance/Healthandsocialcaretopics/Chlamydia/index.htm) and therefore the organism can exist in the patient's system for significant amounts of time (even years) without detection.

OPHTHALMIA NEONATORUM

Any conjunctivitis in a child aged under 21 days is known as ophthalmia neonatorum and is a notifiable disease. Historically, this was because it tended to be caused by gonococci transmitted from the mother in the birth canal. Gonococcal conjunctivitis is very uncommon now, especially as women are screened during pregnancy. Chlamydia infection is much more likely to be the cause at present.

Swabs should be taken from the baby and the health visitor notified for follow-up. Gonococcal conjunctivitis is very purulent and there is a risk of corneal perforation. Chlamydial conjunctivitis tends to be less acute, with only slight stickiness.

SWABS

Other than in neonate and suspected chlamydia infection, there is little point in taking swabs from patients with conjunctivitis.

The procedure is costly, uncomfortable and, except in very occasional cases that should be identified in the clinic, does not change the treatment given to the patient.

REFERENCES

Gigliotti F, Williams WT, Hayden FG (1981). Etiology of acute conjunctivitis in children. *J Pediatr* **98**:531–6.

Miller IM, Wittreich J, Vogel R et al. for the Norfloxacin-Placebo Ocular Study Group (1992). The safety and efficacy of topical norfloxacin compared with placebo in the treatment of acute bacterial conjunctivitis. *Eur J Ophthalmol* **2**:58–66.

Normann EK, Bakken O, Peltola J et al. (2002). Treatment of acute neonatal bacterial conjunctivitis: a comparison of fucidic acid to chloramphenicol eye drops. *Acta Ophthalmol Scand* **80**:183–7.

Rose PW, Harnden A, Brueggemann AB et al. (2005). Chloramphenicol treatment for acute infective conjunctivitis in children in primary care: a randomised double-blind placebo controlled trial. *Lancet* **366**:37–43.

Seal DV, Barrett SP, McGill JI (1982). Aetiology and treatment of acute bacterial infection of the external eye. *Br J Ophthalmol* **66**: 357–60.

Sheikh A, Hurwitz B (2006). Antibiotics versus placebo for acute bacterial conjunctivitis. *Cochrane Database of Systematic Reviews* 2006, Issue 2. Art. No.: CD001211.

Tullo AB, Donnelly D (1995). Conjunctiva. In: Perry JP, Tullo AB (eds), *Care of the Ophthalmic Patient*, 2nd edn. London: Chapman & Hall, 239–52.

Weiss A, Brinser JH, Nazar-Stewart V (1993). Acute conjunctivitis in childhood. *J Pediatr* **122**:10–14.

Wishart PK, James C, Wishart MS (1984). Prevalence of acute conjunctivitis caused by chlamydia, adenovirus, and herpes simplex virus in an ophthalmic casualty department. *Br J Ophthalmol* **68**: 653–5.

Subconjunctival haemorrhage

Spontaneous subconjunctival haemorrhage is a very common presentation. The patient often presents because others have noticed a patch or area of bright blood on the white of the eye.

Subconjunctival haemorrhage can be related to clotting disorders and patients taking aspirin, warfarin or other anti-clotting agents are often prone to haemorrhages of varying severity.

It is always worth checking the blood pressure of patients presenting with this condition. Pitts et al. (1992) found a significant level of undiagnosed hypertension in patients presenting with subconjunctival haemorrhage.

The condition is also associated with Valsalva's manoeuvre – coughing, sneezing or vomiting, for example (Pewitt 2004) or even blowing up balloons (Georgiou et al. 1999).

Some patients experience repeated episodes, perhaps because of a particularly fragile conjunctival blood vessel.

Subconjunctival haemorrhages resolve spontaneously, over variable periods of time that may be protracted if the haemorrhage is severe (perhaps 2 or 3 weeks).

Unless a specific linked factor such as hypertension is discovered, which obviously needs referral to the appropriate physician, treatment consists mainly of education about the cause of the haemorrhage, the possibility of repeat episodes and the nature of self-treatment if it does recur. The patients should also be warned that, because of the potential space underneath the conjunctiva, the blood may spread and the haemorrhage may look worse before it begins to resolve.

The uneven conjunctiva, caused by the bleeding under it, may cause irritation and artificial tears may be helpful.

REFERENCES

Georgiou T, Pearce IA, Taylor RH (1999). Valsalva retinopathy associated with blowing balloons [letter]. *Eye* **13**:686–7.

Pewitt D (2004). What causes haemorrhage? *Rev Optom* **141**:136–7.

Pitts JF, Jardine AG, Murray SB, Barker NH (1992). Spontaneous subconjunctival haemorrhage – a sign of hypertension? *Br J Ophthalmol* **76**:279–99.

14

Section 3

Cornea

Bacterial corneal ulcers

SIGNS AND SYMPTOMS
These are acutely painful red eye, photophobia, blurred vision, increased lacrimation with or without discharge. A white spot on the cornea may be visible to the naked eye.

RISK FACTORS
These are soft contact lens wearers, malnutrition and any other ophthalmic condition in which the corneal epithelium is compromised (Bartlett and Jaanus 2002).

CAUSATIVE FACTORS
The causative factors are lack of hygiene, either with hand washing, contact lens sterilisation or contact lens container, combined with a breakage in the surface of the cornea which is the result of either an abrasion or keratitis from overwear of lenses.

DIAGNOSIS
Slit-lamp examination shows a round white area on the cornea that stains with fluorescein. It may also be associated with stromal infiltrate and anterior chamber activity. An infiltrate refers to an immune response that causes an accumulation of cells or fluid in an area of the body where they do not normally belong.

A corneal scrape is required if the ulcer is > 1–2 mm in diameter (this policy varies between eye units).

CAUSATIVE ORGANISMS
- *Pseudomonas* sp.
- *Acanthamoeba* sp.
- Enterococci.

TREATMENT

Fluoroquinolones are effective against *Pseudomonas* sp. and therefore a good choice of treatment. Either ofloxacin or ciprofloxacin is generally used hourly for 48 h. However, the manufacturer (www.rxmed.com/b.main) and the *British National Formulary* (BMA, RPSGB 2007) advise that Ciloxan must be administered in the following intervals, even during the night:

- On day 1, instil two drops into the affected eye every 15 min for the first 6 h and then two drops into the affected eye every 30 min for the remainder of the day.
- On day 2, instil two drops in the affected eye hourly.
- On days 3–14, place two drops in the affected eye every 4 h. If the patient needs to be treated longer than 14 days, the dosing regimen is at the discretion of the attending physician.

The patient may also need a cycloplegic if there is anterior chamber activity.

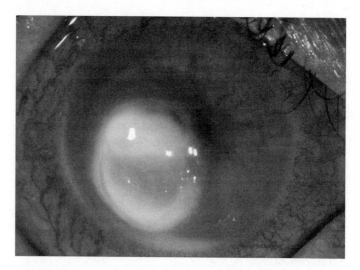

Figure 15.1 *Pseudomonas aeruginosa* corneal ulcer. Reproduced with permission of the Ophthalmic Imaging Department, Flinders Medical Centre, South Australia.

FOLLOW-UP CARE

Review after 48h when the fluoroquinolone has started to become effective. If settling well, then give fluoroquinolone 2 hourly for 2 days and four times daily for a week. Leave contact lenses out for at least a week after finishing eyedrops.

PATIENT EDUCATION

- Explanation of how and why bacterial corneal ulcers occur.
- Stress importance of hand hygiene and sterilisation of contact lenses.
- Wear daily disposable lenses if possible.
- Never leave lenses in overnight even if extended wear.
- Be up for at least an hour in the morning before putting contact lenses in.
- Take lenses out at least an hour before going to bed.
- Maximum 12h wear per day.
- Have a pair of glasses for back-up.
- Give eyes a rest from contact lenses occasionally.

15

OTHER CONTACT LENS PROBLEMS

Keratitis or tiny corneal ulcers can be treated with chloramphenicol, usually 2 hourly for 2 days then four times daily for 5 days if resolving. Patient should still leave lenses out for 2–3 weeks to resolve problems.

Patient education is still very important to prevent bacterial corneal ulcers.

REFERENCES

Bartlett JD, Jaanus SD (2002). *Clinical Ocular Pharmacology*, 4th edn. New York: Butterworth-Heinemann.

British Medical Association, Royal Pharmaceutical Society of GB (2007). *British National Formulary*. London: BMA, RPSGB. Available at: www.rxmed.com/b.main (accessed 1 June 2007).

Bandage contact lenses 16

Bandage contact lenses are soft contact lenses used for therapeutic purposes. They are a crucial aid to the effective management of diseases affecting the external eye. They are a safe, simple, non-surgical treatment used for many conditions affecting the cornea. The contact lens can protect the cornea from exposure or trauma, such as damage caused by trichiasis or abnormalities of the eyelid.

Contact lenses with a low water content can be used to support healing in small corneal perforations or wound leaks (Biswell 2004). Campbell and Koch (2005) also mention the use of bandage contact lenses to stabilise treatment of corneal perforations with cyanoacrylate glue, acting as a barrier between the glue and the movement of the eyelid. As well as protecting the anterior surface of the cornea, bandage contact lenses can also protect a compromised eye in conditions such as a persistent epithelial defect (James et al. 2003) and are a very useful aid to short-term pain management in other conditions such as bullous keratopathy. In such cases these lenses can be difficult to fit, because of the abnormal contour of the corneal surface.

Bandage contact lenses can also provide temporary protection for a severely compromised eye while the patient is awaiting a penetrating keratoplasty. With this treatment improvement can be noted in the eye after local burns or neuroparalytic ophthalmic lesions.

The lenses do not have refractive power (plano) and are available with different sized diameters. The lens may be left in place for weeks or even months, with careful monitoring. Although these lenses can be left in place for prolonged periods, on compromised corneas, with few possible serious adverse events,

Campbell and Koch (2005) stress the need to assess the risks and benefits of the use of therapeutic contact lenses. The benefits include protection of the cornea, pain relief and regeneration of the epithelial layer. The risks include acute corneal hypoxia, resulting from continuous wear of the contact lens, which can potentially lead to iritis. There is also the risk of microbial keratitis.

Bandage contact lenses are a safe and effective method of alleviating symptoms and promoting healing of many ocular surface disorders. The use of a topical antimicrobial, for prophylactic use, is practised in some ophthalmic departments. Biswell (2004) further asserts that such treatment may be required if there are epithelial defects.

These potential risks emphasise the need for high-quality patient education, stressing the need for the patient to seek advice promptly, if any related symptoms occur. The practitioner also needs to reassure patients that they do not have to manage the lens, which is often a concern.

REFERENCES

Biswell R (2004). Cornea. In: Riordan-Eva P, Whitcher J (eds), *Vaughan and Asbury's General Ophthalmology*, 16th edn. London: Lange, 129–53.

Campbell R, Koch T (2005). Indications for contact lens use. In: Krachmer J, Mannis M, Holland E (eds), *Cornea*, 2nd edn. London: Elsevier Mosby, 1309–11.

James B, Chew C, Bron A (2003). *Lecture Notes on Ophthalmology*, 9th edn. London: Blackwell.

Contact lens care

It has become increasingly common practice to use contact lenses to correct refractive error. Benefits to the wearer tend to be sharper, clearer vision, less fogging in damp conditions, better cosmetic effect than spectacles and improved performance for sport and leisure activities. These benefits are conditional on the wearer having a contact lens care regimen that minimises the harmful effects of contact lens use, such as reduced tear film sufficiency, corneal hypoxia, toxic corneal reaction and contact lens-induced infection.

The contact lens-wearing patient presents a challenge for the ophthalmic practitioner because he or she is most likely to come into contact with such a patient when presenting with a contact lens-related problem rather than when all is going well. There are a number of key questions that the clinician should ask in order to make an accurate diagnosis, provide effective treatment and prevent future ophthalmic complications.

WHAT TYPE OF CONTACT LENSES DO YOU WEAR?

Type of lens	Method of use	Issues
Soft daily disposable (hydrogel)	The patient wears one pair and then throws them away No solutions are required	Patients may try to wear lenses for more than one day or sleep in the lenses to save money Patients are not necessarily taught about disinfection of contact lens because it is assumed that they will wear the lenses on only one occasion Hydrogel material is not the most oxygen-permeable material if lenses are worn over extended periods of time (Morgan et al. 2005)
Soft 2-weekly disposable (hydrogel)	The patient wears the lenses for 2 weeks and then throws them away The patient should take the lenses out every night and disinfect them These lenses are often supplied by the optometrist as part of a package with a multi-purpose solution	Patients may overwear their lenses Patients may not dispose of their lenses after 2 weeks Lenses must be disinfected every night Multi-purpose solutions are not always fully effective against a full range of micro-organisms (Hiti et al. 2002, 2005; Borazjani and Kilvington 2005) Hydrogel material is not the most oxygen-permeable material if lenses are worn over extended periods of time (Morgan et al. 2005)
Soft monthly disposable (hydrogel or silicone hydrogel)	The patient wears the lenses for a month and then throws them away The patient should take the lenses out every night and disinfect them These lenses are often supplied by the optometrist as part of a package with a multi-purpose solution or a hydrogen peroxide-based solution	Patients may overwear their lenses – silicone hydrogel lenses have greater oxygen permeability and may be worn for longer periods of time than hydrogel lenses (Morgan et al. 2005) Patients may not dispose of their lenses after 1 month Multi-purpose solutions are not always fully effective against a full range of micro-organisms

Type of lens	Method of use	Issues
Soft extended wear (silicone hydrogel)	High water content lenses for comfort and increased wearing time The patient may keep the lenses in for a month, including wearing the contact lenses overnight No solutions are supplied with these lenses	Infective or toxic reactions can occur on the cornea but reduced corneal sensation may mean that the patient is not aware of the problem Lenses are not taken out and disinfected so that micro-organisms to which the lens is exposed can colonise it
Rigid gas-permeable (hard) and hard lenses	These lenses are not disposable and patients may keep these lenses for 6 months to a year Lenses must be taken out every night These lenses are not always provided as a package with disinfecting solutions and the patient is responsible for buying solutions separately	Lenses can become scratched or damaged, leading to a roughened surface that attracts micro-organisms Damaged lens surface may disturb the integrity of the cornea, leading to increased risk of infection Rigid lenses do not permit diffusion of oxygen to the cornea, making it more vulnerable to infection Solutions are expensive and the patient may try to compromise by re-using solutions or keeping them past their sell-by date (Sobrinho et al. 2003)
Cosmetic lenses (soft)	May be medically prescribed to improve the cosmetic effect of a phthisical eye or an injury Bought to enhance eye colour or give alternative effects May be bought from shops selling novelty lenses; come with instructions and solution but no teaching or education is given to support contact lens use	Usually bought by the young, inexperienced person Not fitted by a trained person No teaching/education given Difficult to insert and remove, leading to trauma to the cornea and risk of infection Cheap disinfecting solutions are supplied that are not necessarily effective against all micro-organisms Lenses may be worn in dry conditions for long periods of time

17

HOW LONG DO YOU WEAR YOUR LENSES EVERY DAY?

This information is important because contact lenses inhibit the blink reflex and the flow of tears across the eye. This results in reduced oxygen supply and reduced exposure to the tear film, which contains lysosomes and enzymes that prevent infection and increased contact time between micro-organisms and the cornea. Different contact lens materials have greater oxygen permeability than others and so appropriate wearing times may vary. In principle the longer the wearing time the more vulnerable the cornea becomes to infection and/or toxic reaction to the contact lens-disinfecting solution, the contact lens material or debris built up on the lens (Morgan et al. 2005).

DO YOU TAKE YOUR CONTACT LENSES OUT BEFORE GOING TO SLEEP?

It is important to elicit this information because sleeping in contact lenses further compromises the blink reflex and flow of tears across the eye; this potentiates the risk of infection or toxic reaction. Wearing of corneal contact lenses also inhibits the corneal response to pain, meaning that a severe reaction can occur before the patient notices the problem particularly, when the lenses are worn overnight (Morgan et al. 2005).

DO YOU EVER BATH, SHOWER, WASH YOUR HAIR OR SWIM IN YOUR CONTACT LENSES?

Acanthamoeba spp. are one-celled protozoa found in tap water and in places where water has dried such as around taps or on bathroom surfaces. They are able to encyst to survive for long periods of time in harsh conditions. Exposure of the contact lens or contact lens case to tap water or acanthamoeba cysts can lead to colonisation of the contact lens cases and surfaces. Once in contact with the corneal stroma *Acanthamoeba* sp. can cause acanthamoeba keratitis, which is notoriously difficult to treat and may be sight threatening (Hiti et al. 2002, 2005; Borazjani and Kilvington 2005).

WHAT TYPE OF SOLUTION DO YOU USE?

There are several types of solution available for the disinfection of contact lenses. A number of studies have indicated that hydrogen peroxide (H_2O_2) 3% two-step solution is the most effective solution for killing most micro-organisms and *Acanthamoeba* spp. in particular.

Multi-purpose solution	Multi-purpose solutions can be used for rubbing, soaking and rinsing contact lenses
	These solutions are the cheapest to buy and are often provided with contact lens care packages by optometrists
	They may contain chemicals such as polyhexamethylene biguanide (PHMB), which are non-toxic to the eye in the concentrations provided in multi-purpose solutions
	These solutions are not always effective in fully eradicating micro-organisms, in particular acanthamoeba cysts and trophozoites (Hiti et al. 2002, 2005; Borazjani and Kilvington 2005)
	For these solutions to work to their **maximum effectiveness**, they **must** be used rigorously as described in the instructions (Guillon and Maissa 2002; Borazjani and Kilvington 2005)
	Some multi-purpose solutions have citrate added to make them more effective in cleaning the surface of the lens of protein deposits and bacteria (Guillon and Maissa 2002)
One-step solution (H_2O_2 3%)	H_2O_2 solution supplied with a catalysing tablet or a contact lens case containing a platinum-neutralising ring
	The contact lens case is filled with H_2O_2. The lenses are placed in the contact lens case with the tablet or platinum ring that works to neutralise the H_2O_2 in about 6 h
	Neutralisation starts immediately the neutralising tablet or ring is placed in the solution. Lenses are not in contact with the H_2O_2 solution for 6 h and therefore some micro-organisms may survive (Hiti et al. 2002, 2005)
H_2O_2 3% two-step solution	H_2O_2 solution supplied with a separate vial of neutralising solution
	The contact lens case is filled with H_2O_2. The lenses are placed in the contact lens case for a minimum of 6 h
	The H_2O_2 is then discarded and the case filled with neutralising solution for 10 min
	This is the gold standard of contact lens disinfection systems shown to eradicate all micro-organisms including *Acanthamoeba* spp.

17

TELL ME HOW YOU CLEAN YOUR CONTACT LENSES?

It is important to recognise that the method of cleaning contact lenses is equally important to the solution used. Regardless of the disinfecting system used, cleaning should be performed regularly and thoroughly, according to manufacturer's instructions, to be effective. If patients do not perform these steps they leave themselves vulnerable to infection.

Action	Rationale
Wash hands before removal and insertion of contact lens Dry hands on a 'fluff-free' towel	To reduce exposure of the eye and lens to contamination Dust and fluff can contaminate the surface of the lens, causing trauma to the cornea and acting as a focus for infection
Rub the surface of the contact lens between thumb and forefinger for at least 10 s on each side If an H_2O_2 system is used a separate enzymatic degreasing solution should also be used If a multi-purpose solution is used a few drops of multi-purpose solution can be used for rubbing There are solutions on the market that contain citrate, which manufacturers claim obviates the need for rubbing the lens (Guillon and Maissa 2002)	This stage is called 'rubbing' and is vital for removing surface deposits from the lens to allow the disinfecting solution to work more effectively Proteins and oil from the tear film collect on the contact lens surface These deposits trap micro-organisms and provide a food source for their survival The protein deposits can themselves cause a toxic response in the cornea and conjunctiva
Soaking times identified on the manufacturer's instructions should be treated as minimum soaking times to ensure adequate disinfection Soaking in a recognised solution appropriate to contact lens type and material	This stage is called the soaking or disinfection stage Soaking times vary according to the type of solution used. Lenses should be exposed to the full-strength solution for the full time identified by the manufacturer Multi-purpose solutions are less effective against a range of microbes and therefore need stricter adherence to the rules of disinfection and cleaning

Action	Rationale
	Solutions only have a shelf-life of 28 days once opened. Keeping solutions for longer may mean that the solution acts as a reservoir for micro-organisms or becomes less effective. Use of the wrong soaking solution for the lens material can lead to damage to the lens surface, resulting in damage to the cornea
Rinse contact lenses either using multi-purpose solution or sterile saline solution	This stage is the rinsing stage. It is vital that chemicals in disinfecting solution are not left in contact with the cornea and conjunctiva because they can set up toxic reaction, leading to irritation, pain, itching and discomfort

HOW OFTEN DO YOU CHANGE YOUR CONTACT LENS CASE?

The contact lens case has been found to be a primary factor in the development of contact lens-related infections. Debris and proteins build up within the contact lens case, leading to the formation of 'biofilm'. Biofilm is impermeable to disinfecting solutions, allowing micro-organisms including *Acanthamoeba* sp. to grow and survive in the case. The contact lenses then become contaminated by biofilm and micro-organisms. Contact lens cases should be changed at least monthly. They should be rinsed in contact lens-disinfecting solution, wiped with a lint-free cloth and left to air dry when not in use (Boost and Cho 2005).

CONCLUSION

Information provided in this chapter is intended to provide an overview of the issues related to the use and care of contact lenses. It is intended for use as a framework to assess the contact lens-wearing patient. There is much research available in the care, disinfection and management of contact lenses and compliance with this. There are many different types of contact lens materials and contact lens solutions; this, coupled with a variety of contact lens care regimens and a rapidly changing commercial environment, means that assessment of the contact lens-wearing patient must be performed on an individual basis in collaboration with the patient's optometrist and using the best available evidence at the time.

REFERENCES

Boost MV, Cho P (2005). Microbial flora of tears of orthokeratology patients, and microbial contamination of contact lenses and contact lens accessories. *Optom Vis Sci* **82**:451–8.

Borazjani RN, Kilvington S (2005). Efficacy of multipurpose solutions against *Acanthamoeba* species. *Contact Lens Anterior Eye* **28**:169–75.

Guillon M, Maissa C (2002). Acceptance of two multipurpose solutions: MPS containing HPMC versus citrate-based MPS without rubbing. *CLAO J* **28**:186–91.

Hiti K, Walochnik J, Haller-Schober EM, Faschinger C, Aspöck H (2002). Viability of *Acanthamoeba* after exposure to a multipurpose disinfecting contact lens solution and two hydrogen peroxide systems. *Br J Ophthalmol* **86**:144–6.

Hiti K, Walochnik J, Faschinger C, Haller-Schober EM, Aspöck H (2005). One- and two-step hydrogen peroxide contact lens disinfection solutions against *Acanthamoeba*: How effective are they? *Eye* **19**:1301–5.

Morgan PB, Efron N, Hil EA, Raynor MK, Whiting MA, Tullo AB (2005). Incidence of keratitis of varying severity among contact lens wearers. *Br J Ophthalmol* **89**:430–6.

Sobrinho M, Vicente de Andrade MD, Carvalho RA (2003). Do the economic and social factors play an important role in relation to the compliance of contact lenses care? *Eye Contact Lens: Sci Clin Pract* **29**:210–12.

17

Corneal scrape

If a patient has a suspected bacterial corneal ulcer it may be necessary to take a corneal scrape, particularly in patients who do not wear contact lenses or if *Acanthamoeba* sp. is suspected.

PROCEDURE
- The usual kit provided by microbiology includes four agar plates: blood agar (COLBA), fastidious anaerobe agar (FAA), chocolate agar (COLCH) and Sabouraud's agar (SABC). It may also contain a small bottle of brain–heart infusion broth, some microscope slides, swabs with transport medium and a sterile pot.
- Before use, check that there are no surface colonies on any of the plates and that the broth is clear.
- Anaesthetise the cornea with oxybuprocaine (Minims Benoxinate) or amethocaine eyedrops.
- Wipe pus, mucus and debris from the ulcer with a sterile swab and send for culture in transport medium.
- Scrape the edge of the base of the ulcer with the angled, sharp flange of a hypodermic needle.
- Gently sweep the surface of the four agar plates using a fresh green needle every time.
- Inoculate the broth with material as aseptically as possible.
- Using another fresh needle deposit some material on to the centre of a glass microscope slide and label with patient's details.
- Ensure that all specimens are adequately labelled and send to microbiology without delay.
- Complete a microbiology request form providing details of whether patient wears contact lenses, querying *Acanthamoeba* sp. and antibiotics prescribed.

- If patient is a contact lens wearer, the lens and solution can be sent for culture.

REPORTING TIMES
A Gram film can be requested urgently and reported on straight away. The rest of the cultures are read at 2 days, then usually daily up to 5–7 days. The acanthamoeba report takes 7 days and the fungal one 5–7 days.

THE KIT
- Blood agar: grows most bacteria
- Chocolate agar (heated blood): grows most bacteria especially *Haemophilus* spp. and respiratory bacteria.
- Sabouraud's agar: specifically fungal
- FAA: more specific to anaerobes
- Broth: for enrichment; boosts numbers of organisms if not enough on plates
- Black charcoal swab: for *Acanthamoeba* sp.
- Glass slide: for Gram staining.

Adapted from Manchester Royal Eye Hospital procedures and the Bournemouth Eye Unit junior doctor handbook.

FURTHER READING
BSOP 52 – National Standards Method, Health Protection Agency (Investigation of intraocular fluid and corneal scrapings). Available at: www.hpa-standardmethods.org.uk

Leck AK, Matheson MM, Heritage J. *A Laboratory Manual and Guide to Management of Microbial Keratitis.* Available at: www.iceh.org.uk/files/suppkeratitis/SK_manual.pdf

18

Corneal topography

19

Computerised corneal topography is used for both investigative and diagnostic analysis. Corneal topography is used to produce an outline of the contour of the corneal surface. There are various systems available commercially, which vary in the methods used to capture information. Thus, despite new technologies, it appears that scales and maps for corneal topography are yet to be standardised.

There is a significant variability between different instruments. Currently, the one most commonly used uses video-keratoscopy and a personal computer (Corbett et al. 1999). This instrument captures a black-and-white image, using a video camera. The method employs the same principles as the Placido disc and keratometer. Placido-based, computerised, video-keratographic, corneal, curvature mapping systems are useful for identifying cases of keratoconus. Although the instruments provide important information in these eyes, they show curvature changes rather than maps of true corneal shape (Rao and Padmanabhan 2000).

By reflecting concentric circles onto the corneal surface, the topography machine captures a keratoscopic image. The mires appear closer together in steeper areas of the cornea and wider apart in the flatter areas. The data are then interpreted through a personal computer. The image provides information that is translated into a topographic colour-coded map (Chang 2004). A good tear film enhances a quality image; conversely, a poor tear film will possibly cause artefacts. The patient should therefore be encouraged to blink before the readings are taken. The procedure is non-invasive.

For optimal vision, it is imperative that the shape, integrity and transparency of the cornea are maintained. The cornea is a significant component in the process of refraction. It is responsible for more than two-thirds of the total refractive power of the eye. Therefore, it is important to identify any changes in the contour of the corneal surface. The corneal curvature is greatest at the centre and smallest at its periphery. The optical performance of the cornea is significantly challenged if the central cornea is flattened below 33 D or steeper than 50 D (Nishida 2005). Corneal mapping looks specifically at the curvature of the cornea and also its dioptric power. The topographic map identifies the steepest and flattest areas of the cornea in each meridian and axis. A colour scale, provided together with the map, provides information to reference the dioptric power of the findings (Kanski 2003). The data are then interpreted through a personal computer.

The findings of corneal topography can assist in the diagnosis of irregularities on the corneal surface caused by keratoconus or astigmatism. It also provides a record of findings that, when repeated in the future, establish whether any changes have occurred in the findings. Changes in the shape of the cornea after surgery, such as corneal graft or cataract extraction, can also be identified (Stollery et al. 2005).

With its increasing popularity, corneal topography is a very important assessment of the corneal status before and after refractive surgery to measure outcomes against the initial findings (Saxena 2003). The visual performance of the postoperative cornea after refractive surgical procedures is dependent on the pupil size; most video-keratoscopes provide pupil-mapping software that depicts the position of the pupil in ambient illumination. This allows interpretations of changes in the topographic map in the region of the pupil, which is more likely to affect visual outcomes (Rao and Padmanabhan 2000).

Topographic maps are a useful visual aid, providing clinicians with pictorial information, helping optimise the information provided for the patient about the condition.

REFERENCES

Chang D (2004). Ophthalmologic examination. In: Riordan-Eva P, Whitcher J (eds), *Vaughan and Asbury's General Ophthalmology*, 16th edn. London: Lange, 29–61.

Corbett M, O'Brart D, Rosen E, Stevenson R (1999). *Corneal Topography*. London: BMJ Books.

Kanski J (2003). *Clinical Ophthalmology: A systematic approach*, 5th edn. London: Butterworth-Heinemann.

Nishida T (2005). Cornea. In: Krachmer J, Mannis M, Holland E (eds), *Cornea: Fundamentals, diagnosis and management*, 2nd edn. London: Elsevier Mosby, 3–26.

Rao S, Padmanabhan P (2000). Understanding corneal topography. *Curr Opin Ophthalmol* **11**:248–59.

Saxena S (2003). *Clinical Practice in Ophthalmology*. New Delhi: Jaypee.

Stollery R, Shaw M, Lee A (2005). *Ophthalmic Nursing*, 3rd edn. London: Blackwell.

Herpes simplex virus (HSV) is a DNA virus that infects only humans. Infection is common; up to 90% of the population are seropositive for HSV-1 antibodies, although most infections are subclinical (Kanski 2003). Herpes simplex keratitis or dendritic ulcers occur as a result of secondary HSV disease or as a recurrence. The primary infection occurs usually in childhood (HSV-1). HSV-2 is mainly genital infection, occurring at 16–30 years of age, but can rarely be transmitted to the eye through infected genital secretions, either sexually or at birth (Kanski 2003). Infection is transferred by contact and the presence of the virus in the bloodstream; when it occurs during the primary infection it induces the production of antibodies that persist throughout life.

MANIFESTATION

Primary infection manifests as herpetic lip lesions, ulcers in the mouth, flu-like symptoms and swollen regional lymph nodes. In immunodeficient patients the symptoms can be severe and they can become quite ill. Primary infection of the eye is less common but can present as unilateral follicular conjunctivitis, lid oedema with vesicular eruptions or ulcerative blepharitis. The patient may also have swollen preauricular lymph glands. Fifty per cent of patients with HSV conjunctivitis develop keratitis after 7–14 days; this may be punctate, dendritic, subepithelial or rarely stromal (Fechner and Teichmann 1998).

Infection of the eye is usually 'back-door' spread to the ophthalmic nerve via the trigeminal ganglion from an orofacial site. It is often difficult to isolate where primary HSV infection manifests as follicular conjunctivitis because it is not common practice to swab every patient with conjunctivitis for viral studies. Indeed

20

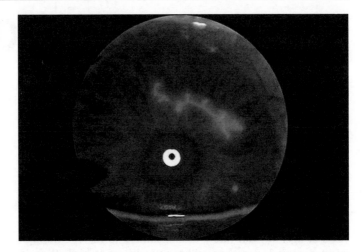

Figure 20.1 Herpes simplex virus.

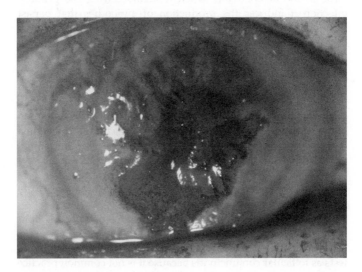

Figure 20.2 Geographic ulcer.

swabbing rarely isolates the virus in any case. For this reason, caution is advised when treating viral conjunctivitis with steroids in case the cause is HSV.

After the primary infection, whether ocular or orofacial, the virus settles in the trigeminal neurons and probably also in the cornea, in a state of latency. The virus maintains a 'dynamic balance' with continuous slow replication of a portion of the viral genome. Recurrence probably comes from neuronal reservoirs and non-neuronal cells such as cornea and skin. Antibodies seem to prevent recurrence of systemic disease but do not influence survival in cells. When the balance between host and virus is disturbed, local recurrence develops. The factors that tend to influence recurrence are illness, stress or anything that lowers the immune system. Bright sun and wind are also thought to be influential in causing recurrence.

Ten per cent of herpetic infections recur within 1 year, 50% within 10 years and >60% within a 20-year observation period (Fechner and Teichmann 1998).

SIGNS AND SYMPTOMS
Patients may complain of red, painful or gritty eyes. They may be photophobic and complain of blurred vision and lacrimation. They may also have a common cold or other illness.

DIAGNOSIS
An accurate diagnosis is made by detailed history taking and slit-lamp examination of the eye. Examination with fluorescein shows either micro-dendrites, which appear star shaped (keratitis), or a larger, more central, 'dendrite'-shaped ulcer. Corneal sensation is usually reduced and there may be some associated stromal infiltrate.

TREATMENT
Most HSV infections will heal spontaneously within 2–3 weeks; however, corneal infections may leave scarring and treatment is aimed at reducing the duration of the infection and minimising corneal scarring. Secondary stromal involvement occurs quite frequently whether or not the infection is treated. Fechner and Teichmann (1998) recommend débriding the viral ulcer carefully

20

with a cotton bud to remove virus particles, but this is not commonly carried out in the UK. Treatment here is usually with antiviral ointment aciclovir (Zovirax) five times a day for 10 days. The ointment does not kill the virus but reduces replication by inhibiting nucleic acid synthesis.

Aciclovir is 30 times more potent against the HSV cell than the host cell and is broken down rapidly by the host cells, thereby causing less damage to the healthy cells (Rang et al. 2003). However, the antiviral ointment can still be quite toxic to the cornea, which can take some weeks to recover. In this situation the addition of lubricants can be beneficial. As aciclovir is quite toxic, its use should be limited to a firm diagnosis of HSV. If there is any doubt it is safer to treat the patient with ocular chloramphenicol or a lubricant and follow up the patient.

It is commonly accepted within complementary medicine circles that taking high doses of vitamin C (1 g/day) can help reduce the duration of the virus (Brewer 2002). However, it is difficult to find actual research to validate these claims; certainly a healthy immune system appears to help prevent recurrence of the virus.

If there is corneal stromal involvement steroid eyedrops may be used in conjunction with aciclovir to reduce the incidence of stromal scarring. This is usually in the form of Predsol eyedrops; however, once steroids have been used any future recurrences tend to need the combined treatment.

Patients should be warned that repeated recurrences of HSV can lead to further scarring and possible reduction in vision, depending on the location of the infection. Central dendritic ulcers are more likely to affect vision than peripheral scarring.

REFERENCES

Brewer S (2002). *Encyclopaedia of Vitamins, Minerals and Herbal Supplements*. London: Constable & Robinson Ltd.

Fechner P, Teichmann K (1998). *Ocular Therapeutics*. Thorofare, NJ: Slack Inc.

Kanski JJ (2003). *Clinical Ophthalmology*, 5th edn. Philadelphia: Butterworth-Heinemann.

Rang H, Dale M, Ritter J, Moore P (2003). *Pharmacology*. Edinburgh: Churchill Livingstone.

20

Marginal ulcers and keratitis

BACKGROUND AND DEFINITION

This is a common disorder thought to be secondary to a hyper-sensitivity reaction to staphylococcal exotoxins – the eye's response to the breakdown products of *Staphylococcus aureus* (Mozayeni and Lam 1998).

It is particularly common in patients who have chronic staphylococcal blepharitis and associated meibomianitis.

SIGNS

- Subepithelial infiltrate of the cornea, usually separated by a clear area of cornea between the ulcer and limbus
- Localised peripheral stromal infiltrates, which tend to occur along the oblique meridians (that is, 2, 4, 8 and 10 o'clock positions)
- The lesion spreads circumferentially, also associated with a breakdown of the epithelium which will stain when fluorescein is instilled
- Within days blood vessels bridge the clear area of cornea, causing neovascularisation of the area
- May or may not have associated anterior chamber inflammation, depending on severity.

SYMPTOMS

Patients usually complain of sore, red, watering, achy eye and may also have an associated conjunctivitis.

These patients may also complain of dry eyes as the tear film is affected by blepharitis and meibomianitis.

TREATMENT

Acute symptoms should be treated with topical steroids and antibiotics, usually Predsol-N four times daily for 1 week then twice daily for 1 week. The steroid dampens down the inflammation and the antibiotic clears the bacterial infection responsible for the reaction. Long-term prevention must be aimed at lid hygiene to clear up the blepharitis and meibomianitis (Newell 1996).

CURRENT THINKING

All adult patients have their intraocular pressure (IOP) checked before steroid therapy as a baseline measure in case of steroid-induced glaucoma.

Steroids are tailed off rather than stopped after a week, so that a rebound inflammation does not occur.

REFERENCES

Mozayeni R, Lam S (1998). Phlyctenular keratoconjunctivitis and marginal staphylococcal keratitis. In: Krachmer J, Mannis M, Holland E, Palay D (eds), *Cornea Text and Color Atlas*, CD-ROM. St Louis, MO: Mosby, Chapter 109.

Newell FW (1996). *Ophthalmology, Principles and Concepts*, 8th edn. St Louis, MO: Mosby.

Recurrent corneal erosion

BACKGROUND
Recurrent corneal erosion (RCE) syndrome is a condition that is characterised by a disturbance at the level of the corneal epithelial basement membrane, resulting in defective adhesions and recurrent breakdowns of the epithelium.

CAUSES
RCE syndrome may occur secondary to corneal injury (often from an animal or vegetable cause – fingernails, plants, etc.) or spontaneously. In the latter case, some predisposing factor, such as diabetes or a corneal dystrophy, may be the underlying cause. Morrison et al. (1998) suggest that there is a high prevalence of recurrent ocular symptoms after traumatic corneal abrasion and many of these patients never re-present to an ophthalmologist, but just cope with their symptoms. They suggest that more thought be given to initial treatment regimens, and long-term follow-up should be undertaken to consider the prevalence of problems.

PHYSIOLOGY
The epithelial healing process begins when basal epithelial cells undergo mitosis, producing new cells that occupy fresh wounds. Basal cells adhere the epithelium to the stroma in two ways: they secrete the basement membrane and they contain hemidesmosomes, which are essentially lynchpins that protrude through the posterior surface of basal cells and into the stroma; each is held in place by an anchoring fibril. Any disruption to basal cell production makes the eye more prone to recurrent erosion.

The primary abnormality with RCE syndrome is poor adhesion of the epithelium to the Bowman membrane as a result of a failure to establish or maintain normal adhesion complexes. Multiple recurrences are common because the basal epithelial cells require at least 8–12 weeks to regenerate or repair the epithelial basement membrane (www.emedicine.com/oph/topic113.htm).

PRESENTATION

The primary symptom of RCE syndrome is mild-to-severe eye pain. Sudden sharp pain is often felt in the early morning during sleep or on awakening, when a frank epithelial defect occurs because of the eyelid movement across the loosened epithelium. The pain may last for only a few seconds but may persist. Commonly, the pain resolves during the day.

Patients who have experienced this may be so worried about the pain on waking – the herald of another bad day – that they are unable to sleep well.

Attacks of pain and ocular irritation occurring in the early morning hours, or upon awakening, are understandable because corneal hydration from lid closure may be a factor affecting epithelial adhesion. Improperly adhered epithelial cells stick preferentially to the lid and are pulled away from the cornea as the lid moves.

Recurrences affect the area of the cornea that was previously injured.

FINDINGS

Depending on the severity of the erosion, corneal examination findings may be totally normal. A classic history of recurrent pain upon awakening is often more important than seeing signs of corneal irregularity in making the correct diagnosis of RCE syndrome.

Epithelial loss may be seen with epithelial microcysts and bullae.

There may be barely visible epithelial irregularity where the erosion has almost healed. There may be pooling around areas of healed and irregular but non-staining epithelium.

RCEs can be classified as either micro- or macroform. With macroform erosions, severe pain persists from hours to days as a result of a large area of the epithelium being separated from the cornea. They are more likely to be associated with a corneal dystrophy.

After trauma, the microform type of erosion always occurs at the site of the original abrasion. Microform recurrent erosions are characterised by intraepithelial microcysts with a minor break in the epithelium. Pain lasts from minutes to hours as the small break heals rapidly (Verma and Ehrenhaus 2007).

PREVENTION

Prevention after corneal abrasion of an animal or vegetable cause, by using ointment at night to lubricate the eye and prevent epithelial loss, is one of the key messages for practitioners and patients. Although Eke et al. (1998) suggested that this may not be a particularly useful idea, it is the only strategy that the practitioner has available that attempts to prevent the syndrome occurring – as it is clear that cure can be difficult and the problem can be painful and distressing and last for a considerable time. In general, the original abrasion is treated with antibiotic ointment four times daily until the epithelium has healed (the patient decides when the eye has stopped being painful) and then at night for the rest of the 28 days for which the tube is current. Further ointment, such as Lacri-Lube or Lubri-Tears, may be suggested for a longer period of time but practitioner experience suggests that this is unlikely to be used!

Explanation of the possibility of RCE syndrome may aid compliance with treatment.

TREATMENT

As episodes tend to occur on waking, it seems to make sense to keep the eye lubricated overnight to prevent epithelial adhesion to the lid. A long-acting ointment is often prescribed at bedtime, for a longer period of time (up to 6 months or longer) to allow adequate time for healing. The use of artificial tears during the day may also be helpful in keeping the eye moist.

Treatment for recurrent erosion that does not settle with conservative treatment includes:

- Bandage contact lenses: for a significant period of time to allow healing and prevent recurrence.
- Medical therapy: patients with recalcitrant recurrent corneal erosions often show increased levels of matrix metalloprotease (MMP) enzymes that dissolve the basement membrane and fibrils of the hemidesmosomes, and lead to the separation of the epithelial layer. Treatment with oral tetracycline antibiotics (such as doxycycline or oxytetracycline) together with a topical corticosteroid (such as prednisolone), reduce MMP activity and may help to resolve the problem and prevent further episodes (Hope-Ross et al. 1994; Dursun et al. 2001; Ramamurthi et al. 2006).
- Autologous serum eyedrops: Geerling et al. (2004) suggest that these help the cornea to heal well without any of the disadvantage of 'foreign' substances and preservatives contained in other ocular lubricants; by nature they are non-allergenic and their biomechanical and biochemical properties are similar to normal tears.
- Alcohol delamination of the epithelium has been suggested (Dua et al. 2006).
- Anterior stromal puncture: this consists of making tiny holes on the surface of the cornea to promote the production of new basement membrane and cause stronger attachments between corneal cells and the underlying substrate (Marechal-Courtois and Duchesne 1993).
- Superficial phototherapeutic keratectomy: with a diamond burr to smooth the basement membrane (Soong et al. 2002) or, more usually, with an excimer laser (Rapuano 1997) – the ablated anterior corneal stromal surface supports stable re-epithelialisation.

REFERENCES

Dua HS, Lagnada R, Raj D et al. (2006). Alcohol delamination of the corneal epithelium: an alternative in the management of recurrent corneal erosions. *Ophthalmology* **113**:404–11.

Dursun D, Kim M, Solomon A, Pflugfelder S (2001). Treatment of recalcitrant recurrent corneal erosions with inhibitors of matrix metalloproteinase-9, doxycycline and corticosteroids. *Am J Ophthalmol* **132**:8–13.

Eke T, Morrison D, Austin DJ (1998). Topical ointment does not prevent recurrent symptoms following traumatic corneal abrasion. *Br J Ophthalmol* **82**:109.

Geerling G, MacLennan S, Hartwig D (2004). Autologous serum eye drops for ocular surface disorders. *Br J Ophthalmol* **88**:1467–74.

Hope-Ross M, Chell P, Kervick G, McDonnell P, Jones H (1994). Oral tetracycline in the treatment of recurrent corneal erosions. *Eye* **8**(Pt 4):384–8.

Marechal-Courtois C, Duchesne B (1993). Recurrent corneal erosion. *Bull Soc Belg Ophtalmol* **247**:13–15.

Morrison D, Eke T, Austin DJ (1998). High prevalence of recurrent symptoms following uncomplicated traumatic cornea. *Br J Ophthalmol* **82**:849.

Ramamurthi S, Rahman M, Dutton G, Ramaesh K (2006). Pathogenesis, clinical features and management of recurrent corneal erosions. *Eye* **20**:635–44.

Rapuano CJ (1997). Excimer laser phototherapeutic keratectomy: long-term results and practical considerations. *Cornea* **16**:151–7.

Soong HK, Farjo Q, Meyer RF (2002). Diamond burr superficial keratectomy for recurrent corneal erosions. *Br J Ophthalmol* **86**:296–8.

Verma A, Ehrenhaus MP (2007). Corneal erosion, recurrent. Available at www.emedicine.com/oph/topic113.htm (accessed 1 June 2007).

Section 4

Angle and aqueous

Acute glaucoma

PRIMARY ACUTE ANGLE-CLOSURE GLAUCOMA

This is a medical emergency. The condition is often misdiagnosed in non-ophthalmic settings as migraine or uveitis and, because of this, can lead to avoidable blindness.

The condition is normally unilateral and the patient presents with the following signs and symptoms: ocular and periorbital pain, and reduced visual acuity; the patient also usually complains of haloes around lights as well as nausea and vomiting resulting from vagal stimulation. The affected eye will be infected (red) and the cornea will be hazy because of oedema; the pupil will be oval, mid-dilated and non-reactive.

Intraocular pressure (IOP) in that eye can be as high as 50–100 mmHg.

MANAGEMENT

There is considerable variation in the details of treatment by different ophthalmologists but the aim of treatment is to reduce IOP, to limit any ischaemic sequelae (Seang-Mei at al. 2003).

- Category orange at triage.
- Intravenous access is essential for the delivery of intravenous acetazolamide (Diamox) 500 mg stat, a carbonic anhydrase inhibitor:

> '**Acetazolamide** ... intravenous injection (intramuscular injections are painful because of the alkaline pH of the solution). It is used as an adjunct to other treatment for reducing intra-ocular pressure. Acetazolamide is a sulphonamide; blood disorders, rashes and other

sulphonamide-related side-effects occur occasionally. It is not generally recommended for long-term use; electrolyte disturbances and metabolic acidosis that occur may be corrected by administering potassium bicarbonate.' (BMA, RPSGB 2007)

Hyperosmotic agents reduce vitreous volume as well as total body fluid reduction through osmotic diuresis.

- Oral acetazolamide 500 mg orally stat, once no longer vomiting.
- An antiemetic such as metoclopramide 10 mg by slow intravenous injection.
- Analgesia is not always required because acetazolamide usually acts quickly to reduce IOP and hence the symptoms.
- Instil pilocarpine 2% only when the IOP is sufficiently lowered (<40 mmHg) because it is ineffective during the acute phase (Kanski 2003). In the initial attack, the elevated pressure in the anterior chamber causes a pressure-induced ischaemic paralysis of the iris. At this time, pilocarpine would be ineffective.
- There is no place in the treatment of acute angle-closure glaucoma for intensive miotic treatment because the parasympathomimetic effects of bradycardia, nausea, vomiting and colic become marked with systemic absorption (Kanski 2003; BMA, RPSGB 2007).
- Pilocarpine 4% can cause shallowing of the anterior chamber by increasing lens axial thickness, so is better avoided.
- Other topical eyedrops used include: β-adrenergic antagonists – β blockers such as timoptol provided that it is not contraindicated; α-adrenergic agonists such as Iopidine. No one β blocker has been found to be more effective than any other.
- An anti-inflammatory such as Pred Forte should be prescribed to reduce any inflammatory activity in the anterior chamber.
- Allowing the patient to lie supine (if able to do so) is of benefit because it can reduce the crowding of the angle by gravity.
- Intravenous 20% mannitol 1–2 g/kg body weight should be commenced but only if the intravenous acetazolamide is not working to lower the IOP.

- Oral 50% glycerol 1 g/kg body weight is given only if intravenous acetazolamide or intravenous mannitol is not working to reduce IOP.
- YAG (yttrium–aluminium–garnet) peripheral iridotomy to affected eye once the inflammation has subsided, normally after 12–24 h, and the other eye is done prophylactically.

REFERENCES

British Medical Association, Royal Pharmaceutical Society of GB (2007). *British National Formulary* 52. Available at: www.rxmed.com/b.main (accessed 1 June 2007).

Kanski JJ (2003). *Clinical Ophthalmology*, 5th ed. London: Butterworth-Heinemann.

Seang-Mei S, Gazzard G, Friedman D (2003). Interventions for angle closure glaucoma. An evidence-based update. *Ophthalmology* **110**: 1869–78.

23

Angle assessment

Gonioscopy is the gold standard of assessment of the angle.

GONIOSCOPY

Definition
Gonioscopy is defined as a procedure that enables the examination of the periphery of the anterior chamber angle.

Indications
- History of suspected angle closure
- History of previous attack of angle closure
- Observation of narrow angle identified by other techniques.
- Blunt trauma with hyphaema when resolved
- Blunt trauma where angle recession is suspected
- Possible anterior chamber neovascularisation
- Recent or previous branch or central vein occlusion
- General glaucoma assessment.

Procedure
Usually carried out with Goldmann mirrored lens; this is described as 'indirect gonioscopy' because the angle is observed as a mirrored image:

- Explain procedure to patient
- Instil topical anaesthetic eyedrops
- Position patient at slit-lamp
- Slit-lamp should be set with high magnification and slit fully open
- Fill the concave surface of the gonioscopy lens with bubble-free fluid such as Celluvisc or Viscotears

- With patient looking straight ahead, insert the lower lip of the lens into the lower fornix and lift the upper lid over the upper lip of the lens; the D-shaped mirror should be put at the 12 o'clock position
- View the angle by gently rotating the lens through 360°
- Remove the lens by parting the eyelids clear of the lens; gently rock the lens back and forth to break the seal; if the lens is firmly attached through capillary vacuum, this can be broken by pressing firmly on the lateral sclera with the tip of a clean finger through the eyelid
- Decontaminate and disinfect the lens.

Structures visible in the anterior chamber

The angle structures from anterior to posterior are:

1. Schwalbe's line which looks like a thin, glistening line and is the termination of Descemet's membrane where the corneal scleral meshwork terminates.

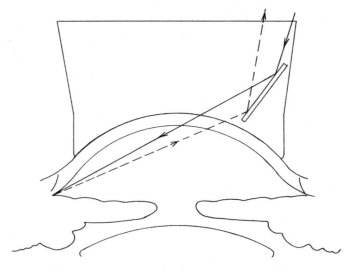

Figure 24.1 Single-mirror gonioscopy lens.

2. The trabecular meshwork, which is a translucent light-grey colour, and darkens with age. The canal of Schlemm may be visible when full of blood (in a soft globe or if excess pressure is applied to the sclera during gonioscopy).
3. Scleral spur which is a protrusion of the sclera into the anterior chamber.
4. Ciliary body band is broader inferiorly and temporally, which may explain why the anterior chamber is wider inferiorly and temporally. The colour in light eyes is grey–white and in dark eyes brown or charcoal grey.
5. Iris processes in some angles, which are fine, lacy fibres or coarse dense network.
6. Blood vessels running in a radial pattern are often seen in normal eyes. Blood vessels running randomly in various directions are likely to be abnormal (Kanski 2003).

There are a number of grading systems used to classify the depth of anterior chamber following gonioscopy, examples being:

- Kolker and Hetherington (1970) system where the widest angles are designated grade 4 through to an occluded angle graded at 0.
- Spaeth's system assesses and grades iris insertion, angle, contour of peripheral iris and pigmentation of posterior trabecular meshwork (Spaeth 1971).
- Shaffer's method (Shaffer 1960) estimates the angle that the iris makes with the ciliary body/trabeculum and correlates well with the van Herrick system.

Generally the angles are described in words in clinical records with any abnormal findings.

OTHER METHODS OF ANTERIOR CHAMBER DEPTH ASSESSMENT

Torchlight examination
Using a torch, shine the light from the temporal side on to the cornea, parallel but anterior to the iris. If you can see a shadow on the nasal limbus, this indicates a narrow angle and shallow

anterior chamber. This is a simple test, which may indicate that caution is needed when dilating the pupil and the patient may be at risk of developing angle closure.

Slit-lamp technique

The central corneal thickness is approximately 0.5 mm. Using a slit-lamp beam the depth of the chamber is estimated. In an average adult eye the accommodation is about 3.15 mm in depth. If it is <2.5 mm the eye is at risk of angle closure.

Van Herrick anterior chamber assessment using a slit-lamp

This test uses a slit beam to compare the depth of the peripheral anterior chamber with the thickness of the cornea. When the depth of the peripheral anterior chamber is less than a quarter of the corneal thickness it is considered shallow (Thomas and Parikh 2006).

Using a full-length slit beam and × 15 magnification, shine the beam at 60° through the anterior chamber with the outer beam on the limbus. Assuming the corneal thickness is 1 unit, assess the depth of the anterior chamber from corneal endothelium to iris. The van Herrick test has been found to be a poor predictor of an occludable angle (Thomas et al. 1996). Grade 4 and 5 angles may close and grades 0–2 may not! Both torchlight and van Herrick's tests detect occludable angles, which are a risk factor only for angle closure. Only a minority of occludable angles progress to angle closure. The van Herrick test for screening on its own will result in too many false positives (Thomas and Parikh 2006).

Grade	Ratio of aqueous gap/cornea	Clinical interpretation	Shaffer angle (°)
4	$>\frac{1}{2}$:1	Closure impossible	45–35
3	$\frac{1}{2}-\frac{1}{4}$:1	Closure impossible	35–20
2	$\frac{1}{4}$:1	Closure possible	20
1	$<\frac{1}{4}$:1	Closure likely with full dilatation	≤10
0	Nil	Closed	0

From Barnard (1999/2000).

These three methods of anterior chamber assessment are fairly approximate; gonioscopy is recognised as being the gold standard and is recommended by the European Glaucoma Society (2003) as a fundamental part of the comprehensive eye examination for patients with suspected glaucoma.

REFERENCES

Barnard S (1999/2000). *Assessment of the Anterior Chamber*. London: City University. Available at: www.academy.org.uk/lectures/barnard12.htm (accessed 17 October 2007).

European Glaucoma Society (2003). *Terminology and Guidelines for Glaucoma*, 11th edn. London: European Glaucoma Society.

Kanski JJ (2003). *Clinical Ophthalmology*, 5th edn. Philadelphia: Butterworth-Heinemann.

Kolker AE, Hetherington J (1970). Clinical interpretation of gonioscopic findings. In: *Becker-Shaffer's Diagnosis and Therapy of the Glaucomas*, 3rd edn. St Louis, MO: Mosby, 41–50.

Shaffer RN (1960) Primary glaucomas. Gonioscopy, ophthalmoscopy, and perimetry. *Trans Am Acad Ophthalmol Otolaryngol* **64**:112–27.

Spaeth GL (1971). The normal development of the human anterior chamber angle: a new system of descriptive grading. *Trans Ophthalmol Soc UK* **91**:709–39.

Thomas R, Parikh RS (2006). How to assess a patient for glaucoma. *Community Eye Health J* **19**:36–7.

Thomas R, George T, Muliyil J (1996). The flashlight and van Herrick's test are poor predictors of occludable angles. *Aust N Z J Ophthalmol* **24**:251–6.

24

Tonometry

The measurement of intraocular pressure (IOP) is based on the Imbert–Fick principle:

> . . . in an ideal, dry thin-walled sphere, the pressure inside the sphere (P) is equal to the force necessary to flatten the surface (F) divided by the area of flattening (A) calculated, thus: $P = F/A$.

In the eye, the cornea is flattened and IOP is determined by measuring the applanating force and the area flattened. The force necessary to flatten the cornea is converted to millimetres of mercury by multiplying the grams by 10.

Other methods of IOP measurements include:

- 'Air puff' non-contact tonometer, which uses a pulsed jet of air to deform the corneal apex. This method carries less risk of cross-infection and is useful in mass screening. This is less accurate than Goldmann tonometry but Kumar et al. (2006) found that it was within reasonable limits and an acceptable screening method.
- Tonopen: a light portable instrument with an in-built software that automatically self-calibrates after each use and selects the acceptable measurements. It is slightly less accurate than the Goldmann tonometry, although van der Jagt and Jansonius (2005) found that this was within reasonable limits.
- Schiøtz tonometer: this is rarely used in developed countries but is of great value in the developing world. A preset weight is placed on the tonometer, which is then placed on the anaesthetised cornea. The amount that the plunger sinks is measured off the scale and the reading is converted to millimetres

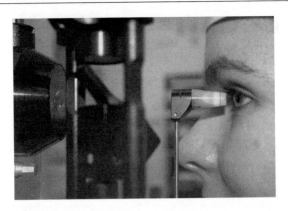

Figure 25.1 Tonometry.

of mercury from a conversion table. This can be used only on a recumbent patient.

- The 'Perkins' tonometer: a hand-held tonometer that is based on the same principle as the Goldmann tonometer.

PROCEDURE FOR GOLDMANN TONOMETRY (FROM SHAW 2006)

The Goldmann tonometer consists of two main parts: (1) a small Perspex cylinder that is applied to the eye by (2) a lever attached to a coiled spring; the tension is controlled by a calibrated drum at the side of the instrument. It is used together with a slit-lamp. Care must be taken when handling the tonometer to avoid damage to the spring-loaded device. It is good practice to calibrate the tonometer before each clinic or at the very least weekly to ensure accurate intraocular measurement. Any defective tonometer (>2 mmHg on calibration) must be sent away for repair.

METHOD

- A clear, concise explanation is given to the patient to ensure cooperation.

- Contact lenses should be removed and Minims lidocaine/fluorescein or proxymetacaine/fluorescein drops instilled into each eye.
- The use of disposable prisms or prism covers is good practice to minimise the spread of infections. Multi-use prisms should be sterilised appropriately between patients and enough prisms should be available to ensure that sterilisation is effective.
- The prism should be placed in the clip at the end of the tonometer arm. During the attachment of the prism, the lever should be supported with a finger to minimise damage to the spring lever.
- The tonometer calibration arm is turned to 1 so that the arm is exerting a slight forward pressure.
- The complete tonometer is placed on the mounting plate on the viewing arm of the slit-lamp and the slit-lamp magnification is set to 10× with a blue filter in place.
- The illuminating arm of the slit-lamp is placed at an angle of 60° to the slit-lamp.
- The patient should be instructed to look straight ahead and the slit-lamp advanced until a bright blue hue is seen just before touching the apex of the cornea. Up to this point it is best observed using the naked eye from the side.
- Looking down the viewing piece of the slit-lamp microscope, the tonometer prism is brought gently into contact with the cornea. Two half-circles are seen through the tonometer, adjacent to each other. The two half-circles must be symmetrically placed on the apex of the cornea. It is important that the slit-lamp be pulled slightly away from the cornea should any fine adjustment be needed. This is to minimise any corneal epithelial damage.
- The calibrated wheel is turned until the half-circles just overlap.
- The IOP is read when the inside edges of the half-circles are just touching.

The IOP in the individual varies over the course of a day (diurnal variation) and patients may need a series of readings, taken over

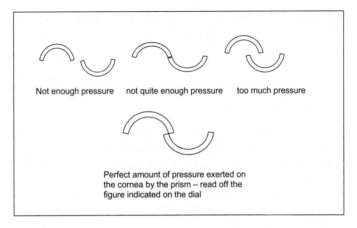

Not enough pressure   not quite enough pressure   too much pressure

Perfect amount of pressure exerted on
the cornea by the prism – read off the
figure indicated on the dial

Figure 25.2 Correct placement of mires when undertaking applanation tonometry.

25

the course of a day (day phasing), to determine the range of pressures particular to the eyes.

REFERENCES
Kumar S, Middlemiss C, Bulsara M et al. (2006). Telemedicine-friendly, portable tonometers: an evaluation for intraocular pressure screening. *Clin Exp Ophthalmol* **34**:666–70.
Shaw M (2006). The angle and aqueous. In: Marsden J (ed.), *Ophthalmic Care*. Chichester: Wiley. p420–460.
van der Jagt LH, Jansonius NM (2005). Three portable tonometers, the TGDc-01, the ICARE and the Tonopen XL, compared with each other and with Goldmann applanation tonometry. *Ophthal Physiol Opt* **25**:429–35.

Section 5

Lens

Biometry (IOL calculation)

The calculation of the power of the intraocular lens implant (IOL) used during cataract surgery is probably the most critical component of the preoperative assessment process for cataract surgery. It directly affects the visual outcome for the patient.

Although the technicalities of the biometry equipment used in the calculation of IOL power may differ between ophthalmic units, the principles of measurement are essentially the same.

Accurate axial length and corneal curvature data allow calculation of the lens power required to focus light on to the retina for effective vision. If the refractive power of the cornea is known, its focal length can be calculated. When the length of the eye is also measured, the difference between the two can be calculated, and a lens chosen to provide the refractive power needed to place the focal point on the retina.

There are various mathematical formulae used in the calculation of IOL powers, a common example being the SRK 1, developed in 1988 by Sanders, Retzlaff and Kraff (Woodcock et al. 2004), which uses the initial refractive properties of the lens (known as the A constant) as a starting point for the calculation:

A constant (2.5 × axial length + 0.9 × corneal curvature) = lens power in dioptres.

This formula is straightforward and therefore the accurate lens predictions should be straightforward – there are confounding factors at all stages of measurement that must be taken into account.

AXIAL LENGTH MEASUREMENTS

These are taken using A-scan ultrasound techniques. As the ultrasound waves pass through the eye, the pulsed echoes from the structures within the eye are reflected and stored within the biometry machine, enabling highly accurate calculation of the axial length measurement.

There really is little room for any margin of error when performing biometry. Inaccurate measurements will lead to unexpected, if not unacceptable, postoperative refractive errors, and in some cases may necessitate removal of the implanted IOL and replacement with an IOL of more appropriate/tolerable power. Woodcock et al. (2004) showed that an error of only 200 μm in a measurement of 25 mm will reduce the patient's outcome by one line of Snellen acuity. They also showed a high level of axial length inaccuracy.

There are two methods of measuring axial length: contact/applanation ultrasonography and non-contact partial coherence laser interferometry (PCLI).

Contact/applanation biometry

This uses a hand-held probe in contact with the patient's corneal surface. Ultrasound pulses are sent though the eye and the time taken for echoes to reach the probe recorded and translated into distance.

- Anaesthetic is required and contact increases the risk of damage to the epithelium and infection (Nemeth et al. 2003).
- Pressure on the cornea will affect readings.
- Patient cooperation is required.
- The presence of silicone oil in the eye gives an artificially low lens prescription as a result of its high density and must be compensated for by the operator.
- Inexperienced operators have poorer results (Findl et al. 2003) and this may be a result of inexperience in the technique, less ability to compensate in complex situations and also reduced patient compliance if the procedure is lengthy.

Partial coherence laser interferometry

Non-contact PCLI methods (commonly the Zeiss IOLMaster) have advantages over the user-dependent ultrasound methods:

- They require no contact with the eye so there is less potential for distortion and damage.
- Reduced operator proficiency still produces good results (Kielhorn et al. 2003).

However, this system is unable to measure axial length in around 17% of eyes (Tehrani et al. 2003) as a result of poor fixation and a degree of lens opacity with which the contact biometry has no problems.

As both systems appear to be required in any eye unit, training and audit are important to ensure good outcomes and all operators, from whatever discipline, must be trained and educated to the same standards to ensure good outcomes for patients. Operators must understand the sources of error and be able to calibrate and adapt the machines.

MEASUREMENT OF THE CURVATURE AND REFRACTIVE POWER OF THE CORNEA – KERATOMETRY

This involves taking measurements of the dimensions of the cornea. Nowadays automated keratometers make this task relatively simple – as long as the operator is trained and experienced in the use of the equipment.

As most corneal surfaces are not spherical, but have both a steeper and a flatter axis, measurement of corneal refractive power must be an average of the two dioptric powers (Woodcock et al. 2004).

If axial length is measured with ultrasound systems, a separate hand-held keratometer is often used and must be held exactly vertical. If PCLI is used, keratometry is integral to the process.

It was initially felt that the use of auto-keratometers was easy, reliable and accurate (Noonan et al. 1998); however, there has been found to be statistically different readings between hand-held and other devices. Rah et al. (2002), Lam et al. (2004) and

Goel et al. (2004) state that the use of keratometry, even with the 'user-independent' IOLMaster, requires operator skill and training to achieve reliable results.

Factors affecting keratometry

- Operator training.
- The use of artificial tears reduces accuracy (Lam et al. 2004).
- Dilating drops change corneal dimensions (Heatley and Whitefield 2002).
- Applanation tonometry affects corneal dimension and axial length measurement if undertaken on the same day as biometry (George et al. 2006).
- Gonioscopy has the same effect (George et al. 2006).
- The use of contact lenses affects corneal dimensions, especially rigid ones (Walline et al. 2004) – contact lenses must be removed before biometry.
- The patient's anatomy may not be in line with the constants in the biometry machinery, which assume a particular model. Corneal refractive power is a function of corneal density, thickness and posterior curvature – pachymetry (measurement of corneal thickness) can be used to modify calculations.
- Any refractive surgery results in difficulty in predicting the IOL required for a good outcome (Wang et al. 2003; Schafer et al. 2005).
- The use of pachymetry probes on the cornea can also reduce corneal thickness and distort results (Rainer et al. 2002).

The final product following biometry readings is a printout detailing a range of IOL powers and corresponding refractive errors, enabling the surgeon to predict accurately and select the IOL that would give the best visual acuity (or refractive results postoperatively), suited to individual patient needs. However, even good measurements can be corrupted by poor manipulation and the simplistic calculation formulae, assuming a perfect and generic patient, have been supplanted by more complex ones (Wang et al. 2003).

Audit data produced by individual units looking at biometry data, predicted and actual outcomes and the type of IOL used can be used to generate modified *A* constants for specific units – this will, if undertaken correctly, tend to produce more accurate results (Gale et al. 2006).

REFERENCES

Findl O, Kriechbaum K, Sacu S et al. (2003). Influence of operator experience on the performance of ultrasound biometry compared to optical biometry before cataract surgery. *J Cataract Refract Surg* **29**:1950–5.

Gale R, Saha N, Johnston R (2006). National Biometry Audit 2. *Eye* **20**:25–8.

George M, Kuriakose T, DeBroff B, Emerson J (2006). The effect of gonioscopy on keratometry and corneal surface topography. *BMC Ophthalmol* **6**:26.

Goel S, Chu C, Butcher M, Jones C, Bagga P, Kotta S (2004). Laser vs ultrasound biometry – a study of intra- and interobserver variability. *Eye* **18**:514–18.

Heatley C, Whitefield L (2002). Effect of pupil dilation on the accuracy of the IOLMaster. *J Cataract Refract Surg* **28**:1993–6.

Kielhorn I, Rajan M, Tesha P, Subryan V, Bell J (2003). Clinical assessment of the Zeiss IOLMaster. *J Cataract Refract Surg* **29**:518–22.

Lam A, Chan R, Chiu R (2004). Effect of posture and artificial tears on corneal power measurements with a handheld automated keratometer. *J Cataract Refract Surg* **30**:645–52.

Nemeth J, Fekete O, Pesztenlehrer N (2003). Optical and ultrasound measurement of axial length and anterior chamber depth for intraocular lens power calculation. *J Cataract Refract Surg* **29**:85–8.

Noonan C, Rao G, Kaye S, Green J, Chandna A (1998). Validation of a handheld automated keratometer in adults. *J Cataract Refract Surg* **24**:411–14.

Rah M, Jackson J, Jones L, Barr J (2002). Comparison of manual keratometry and simulated keratometry readings with corneal topography before and after overnight orthokeratology. American Academy of Optometry. The Cochrane Central Register of Controlled Trials (CENTRAL) 2006 Issue 2.

Rainer G, Petternel V, Findl O et al. (2002). Comparison of ultrasound pachymetry and partial coherence interferometry in the measurement of central corneal thickness. *J Cataract Refract Surg* **28**:2142–5.

Schafer S, Kurzinger G, Spraul W, Kampmeier J (2005). Comparative results of keratometry with three different keratometers after LASIK. *Klin Monatsbl Augenheilk* **22**:419–23.

Tehrani M, Krummenauer F, Blom E, Dick B (2003). Evaluation of the practicality of optical biometry and applanation ultrasound in 253 eyes. *J Cataract Refract Surg* **29**:741–6.

Walline J, Jones L, Mutti D, Zadnik K (2004). A randomized trial of the effects of rigid contact lenses on myopia progression. *Arch Ophthalmol* **122**:1760–6.

Wang L, Misra M, Koch D (2003). Peripheral corneal relaxing incisions combined with cataract surgery. *J Cataract Refract Surg* **29**: 712–22.

Woodcock M, Shah S, Smith R (2004). Recent advances in customising cataract surgery. *BMJ* **328**:92–6.

26

Section 6

Vitreoretinal

Age-related macular degeneration

BACKGROUND

There are two main types of age-related macular degeneration (AMD): neovascular (or wet) AMD, which is characterised by the development of choroidal neovascularisation (CNV), and non-neovascular (or dry) AMD. Non-neovascular AMD makes up approximately 80% of the people with AMD and as yet there are no treatments, but it is less severe and does not cause vision loss to the extent that neovascular AMD does.

There is no proven therapy that prevents the development of AMD, nor unfortunately is there any treatment for dry AMD, although there is evidence suggesting that food supplements containing vitamins, minerals and carotenoids, such as lutein, zeaxanthin and β-carotene, can help slow the progression of AMD (AREDS Research Group 2001; Richer et al. 2004). There are treatments available for wet AMD but they must be applied promptly to prevent growth and leakage of the CNV before scarring of central vision occurs. Currently, on the NHS there are two scientifically proven treatments for wet AMD: laser photocoagulation and photodynamic therapy.

Laser photocoagulation has been in use for many years. Most of the trial evidence for its effectiveness was collected in the late 1980s and early 1990s (Macular Photocoagulation Study Group 1991). However, it is only suitable for a small percentage of patients with small juxta- or extrafoveal lesions (>199 μm from the foveal avascular zone) because it induces an immediate blind or dark spot in the visual field that is not well tolerated by patients with subfoveal CNV lesions.

Photodynamic therapy (PDT) is a two-step procedure carried out in outpatients. First there is an intravenous infusion of a light-

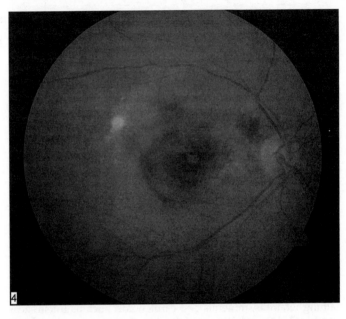

Figure 27.1 Age-related macular degeneration. (Reproduced with permission of the National Institute for Eye Health.)

sensitive drug (verteporfin) and then activation of the drug using a low-power, non-thermal diode laser (689 nm) to the affected area of the macula 15 min after the start of the verteporfin infusion which takes 83 s. Results of the randomised clinical trial (Treatment of AMD with PDT [TAP] Study Group 1999) demonstrated significant benefits for stabilisation of visual loss and lesion growth, preservation of contrast sensitivity and prevention of leakage from the CNV, all important contributors to preservation of a patient's ability to maintain independence.

In recent years there have been significant advances in the development of new pharmacological treatment using a variety of biological targets – namely drugs that target the vascular endothelial growth factor (VEGF). This is the proinflammatory polypeptide that stimulates endothelial growth and thus the development of CNV in the retina. Both pegaptanib sodium (Gragoudas et al. 2004) and ranibizumab (Heier 2005) are anti-VEGF preparations that target vascular endothelial proliferation and inhibit blood vessel growth. They are administered as intra-vitreal injections into the vitreous chamber of the eye every 4–6 weeks and are currently under trial. Preliminary data are very promising because not only have patients maintained vision but also some have improved. The National Institute for Health and Clinical Excellence (NICE) is expected to report favourably on the use of anti-VEGF therapy in the near future.

CONSIDERATIONS FOR NURSES OF RECURRENT NHS TREATMENT: PDT

- Although increased age is the principal risk factor, epidemiological studies highlight other potential risk factors associated with AMD, including cigarette smoking (Mitchell et al. 1999; Pieramici and Bressler 1998; AREDS Research Group 2001). So health education is vital.
- The greatest benefits can be achieved if the diagnosis is made early and patients receive therapy before the lesions become too large or cause too much destruction of the retina, so fast referral systems need to be in place (NICE 2003).
- Patients needing PDT should be warned about the possible side effects that they may experience during infusion, especially low back pain, and the risks of photosensitivity for 48 h after treatment and how to take precautions (see summary of product characteristics enclosed with drug vial for full details).
- Delivery of PDT needs to be accurately timed to ensure that optimum selectivity of the verteporfin is correct (TAP Study Group 1999). This requires the verteporfin to be delivered using a 'syringe driver' set at a rate of 180 mL/h to deliver the 30 mL of reconstituted drug in 10 min. Then the 689 nm laser light should be directed over the CNV and fired at 15 min after the start of the infusion and no later than 20 min after. This ensures that the maximum amount of drug is bound to the high-density lipoprotein (HDL) receptors within the vessel

walls of the CNV. If delivered too early or too late there is a risk of occluding healthy retinal or choroidal vessels.
- PDT is not a single treatment therapy, so the patients should be educated on the need to attend every 12 weeks for possible further treatments.

REFERENCES

AREDS Research Group (2001). Report No 8. A randomised, placebo controlled clinical trial of high dose supplementation with vitamins C and E, beta carotene, and zinc for age-related macular degeneration and vision loss. *Arch Ophthalmol* **119**:1417–36.

Gragoudas ES, Adamis AP, Cunningham AP et al. (2004). Pegaptanib for neovascular age-related macular degeneration. *N Engl J Med* **351**:2805–16.

Heier J (2005). One year data from the ANCHOR study, Anti-VEGF antibody for the treatment of predominantly classic choroidal neovascularisation in AMD. Presented at the American Society of Retinal Specialists, 18 July 2005.

Macular Photocoagulation Study Group (1991). Subfoveal neovascular lesions in age related macular degeneration. Guidelines for evaluation and treatment in the Macular Photocoagulation Study. *Arch Ophthalmol* **109**:1242–57.

Mitchell P, Chapman S, Smith W (1999). Smoking is a major cause of blindness. *Med J Austral* **171**:173–4.

National Institute for Clinical Excellence (2003). *Guidance on the Use of Photodynamic Therapy for Age-related Macular Degeneration.* Technology Appraisal 68. London: NICE.

Pieramici DJ, Bressler SB (1998). Age-related macular degeneration and risk factors for the development of choroidal neovascularization in the fellow eye. *Curr Opin Ophthalmol* **9**:38–46.

Richer S, Stiles W, Statkute L et al. (2004). Double-masked, placebo-controlled, randomized trial of lutein and antioxidant supplementation in the intervention of atrophic age-related macular degeneration: the Veterans LAST study (Lutein Antioxidant Supplementation Trial). *Optometry* **75**:216–30.

Treatment of Age-related Macular Degeneration with Photodynamic Therapy (TAP) Study Group (1999). Photodynamic therapy of subfoveal choroidal neovascularisation in age-related macular degeneration with verteporfin. *Arch Ophthalmol* **117**:1329–45.

Fluorescein angiography

Fluorescein angiography is a diagnostic test that is universally employed throughout the world to detect leakage or damage to the blood vessels of the retina and choroid.

Fluorescein sodium is a highly fluorescent chemical compound synthesised from the petroleum derivatives resorcinol and phthalic anhydride (Jacobs 1992). It absorbs blue light, with peak absorption and excitation occurring at wavelengths between 465 and 490 nm. Fluorescence occurs at the yellow–green wavelengths of 520–530 nm. Although commonly referred to as fluorescein, the dye used in angiography is fluorescein sodium, the sodium salt of fluorescein.

The normal adult dosage is 500 mg injected intravenously. It is typically packaged in doses of 5 mL 10% or 2 mL 25%. On entering the circulation, approximately 80% of the dye molecules bind to serum protein. The remaining unbound or free fluorescein molecules fluoresce when excited with light of the appropriate wavelength. The dye is metabolised by the kidneys and is eliminated through the urine within 24–36 hours of administration. During this period of metabolism and elimination, fluorescein has the potential to interfere with clinical laboratory tests that use fluorescence as a diagnostic marker (Palestine 1991). To avoid any false readings, it may be prudent either to schedule clinical lab tests before the angiogram or to postpone the test for a day or two to allow sufficient elimination of the dye.

SIDE EFFECTS

Side effects of intravenous fluorescein include discoloration of the urine for 24–36 hours and a slight yellow skin discoloration that fades within a few hours. Nursing mothers should be cautioned that fluorescein is also excreted in human milk (Mattern and Mayer 1990). Although there are no known risks or adverse reactions associated with pregnancy, most practitioners will avoid performing fluorescein angiography in pregnant women, especially in their first trimester (Halperin et al. 1990).

Fluorescein is well tolerated by most patients, but angiography is an invasive procedure with an associated risk of complications or adverse reactions. Adverse reactions occur in 5–10% of patients and can range from mild to severe. Transient nausea and occasional vomiting are the most common reactions and require no treatment. These mild reactions seem to be related to the volume of dye and the rate of injection. A relatively slow rate of injection often reduces or eliminates this type of reaction.

Extravasation of fluorescein dye during the injection can be a serious complication of angiography. With a pH of 8–9.8, fluorescein infiltration can be quite painful. Sloughing of the skin, localised necrosis, subcutaneous granuloma and toxic neuritis have been reported after extravasation of fluorescein. With proper injection technique, these complications can usually be avoided.

More severe reactions are rare, but include hives, laryngeal oedema, bronchospasm, syncope, anaphylaxis, myocardial infarction and cardiac arrest (Berkow et al. 1997). Although life-threatening reactions during angiography are rare, Yannuzzi et al. (1986) estimated the risk of death following fundus fluorescein angiography to be 1:222000; the angiographic facility should be properly equipped and prepared to manage serious reactions to the procedure.

CONSIDERATIONS FOR NURSES

- A common misconception, often passed on to patients, is that it is a 'vegetable dye' rather than a synthesised one. Fluorescein contains no iodine and is therefore safe to use in patients known to be allergic to iodine.
- As a result of the risk of anaphylaxis, emergency equipment should be in close proximity to where the procedure is to be carried out.
- Injecting the dye into a distant, small, tortuous vein slowly will produce a poor quality angiogram. It is best to choose a large vein and give a rapid bolus of the dye (Chopdar 1996).

- There is no evidence that fluorescein sodium has any effect on the patient's blood pressure but flashes of bright light on the retina during angiography can result in vagal stimulation, causing a drop in blood pressure and bradycardia.
- If a patient is suspected of having an allergy it may be advisable to do an allergy test: give 0.1 mL 20% fluorescein diluted with 2 mL physiological or 0.9% saline. Observe the patient for 5 min for any untoward reaction (Chopdar 1996).

REFERENCES

Berkow JW, Flower RW, Orth DH, Kelley JS (1997). *Fluorescein and Indocyanine Green Angiography*, 2nd edn. San Francisco, CA: American Academy of Ophthalmology, 7.

Chopdar A (1996). *Fundus Fluorescein Angiography*. London: Butterworth-Heinemann.

Halperin LS, Olk RJ, Soubrane G, Coscas G (1990). Safety of fluorescein angiography during pregnancy. *Am J Ophthalmol* **109**:563–6.

Jacobs J (1992) Fluorescein sodium – what is it? *J Ophthal Photography* **14**:62.

Mattern J, Mayer PR (1990). Excretion of fluorescein into breast milk [letter]. *Am J Ophthalmol* **109**:598.

Palestine AG (1991). Does intravenous fluorescein interfere with clinical laboratory testing? *J Ophthal Photography* **13**:27–8.

Yannuzzi LA, Roher KT, Tindel LJ, Sobel RS, Costanza MA (1986). Fluorescein angiography complication survey. *Ophthalmology* **93**:611–17.

28

Indocyanine green angiography

29

Indocyanine green angiography is a diagnostic test that has recently become more widely used. The dye is used to detect leakage or damage to the blood vessels of the retina and deep choroidal vessels.

Indocyanine green is a highly fluorescent chemical; it is green in colour and fluoresces with visible infrared light. It requires a special digital camera sensitive to these light rays. Indocyanine green angiography has only recently become a practical technique because these cameras have become available relatively recently (Bailey Freund et al. 1997).

The normal adult dosage is 25 mg diluted in 5 mL sterile water.

Indocyanine green is a sterile, water-soluble, tricarbocyanine dye with a peak spectral absorption and emission at 800–810 nm in blood or plasma. It contains about 5% sodium iodide. Transmission of energy by the pigment epithelium is more efficient than in visible light. As the dye is almost 98% bound to proteins, there is minimal leakage of dye from the choroidal vessels, which is why angiography is used in the choroid. Outside ophthalmic use, it is used to determine cardiac output, liver function and liver blood flow.

SIDE EFFECTS AND CAUTIONS

Nursing mothers should be cautioned that it is not known if this dye could be excreted in breast milk. Although there are no known risks or adverse reactions associated with pregnancy, most practitioners will avoid performing indocyanine green angiography in pregnant women, especially in their first trimester.

Indocyanine green is well tolerated by most patients, but angiography is an invasive procedure with an associated risk of complications or adverse reactions. Adverse reactions occur in 0.3%

29

of patients and can range from mild to severe. Symptoms reported include restlessness and urticaria (Hope-Ross et al. 1994).

More severe reactions are rare, but include tachycardia, hypotension and breathlessness, as well as anaphylaxis. Although life-threatening reactions during angiography are rare, Regillo (1999) estimated the risk of death after indocyanine green angiography to be 1:300000. Therefore the angiographic facility should be properly equipped and prepared to manage serious reactions to the procedure.

CONSIDERATIONS FOR NURSES

Indocyanine green angiography is a technique that can provide images of the choroidal vessels through mildly thick blood and serous fluid. It also is possible to use indocyanine green in conjunction with fluorescein angiography in difficult cases (Donald et al. 1998).

- Check any sensitivity to iodine before administration.
- As a result of the risk of anaphylaxis, emergency equipment should be in close proximity to where the procedure is carried out and staff should be trained to use it.
- Injecting dye into a distant, small, tortuous vein slowly will produce a poor quality angiogram. It is best to choose a large vein and give a rapid bolus of the dye (Chopdar 1996).

REFERENCES

Bailey Freund K, Yannuzzi LA, Orlock DA (1997). Ophthalmic fluorescein and indocyanine green angiography: technique and interpretation. Available at www.vrmny.com/angiography.htm (accessed 3 August 2006).

Chopdar A (1996). *Fundus Fluorescein Angiography*. London: Butterworth-Heinemann.

Donald S, Fong MPH, William E et al (1998). Indocyanine green angiography. Ophthalmic technology assessment. *Ophthalmology* **105**:1564–9.

Hope-Ross M, Yannuzzi LA, Gragoudas, ES et al. (1994). Adverse reactions due to indocyanine green. *Ophthalmology* **101**:529–33.

Regillo CD (1999). The present role of indocyanine green angiography in ophthalmology. *Curr Opin Ophthalmol* **10**:189–96.

29

Intravitreal injection procedures in the treatment of AMD

Intravitreal injections are performed to administer a drug directly into the eye (intraocular). Age-related macular degeneration (AMD) is a devastating eye condition that was discussed earlier in this section and there are a number of new treatments that are administered by direct injection into the eye.

Anti-VEGF (anti-vascular endothelial growth factor) agents are administered in order to treat damage to the retina, when the damage has been caused by the growth of abnormal blood vessels growing and leaking fluid and blood products into the eye. This happens primarily in AMD but may occur in other conditions.

New vessel growth and leakage contribute to the progression of AMD and the reduction of patients' quality of life because AMD sufferers find great difficulty in carrying out activities of daily living such as reading, watching television and recognising faces. The loss of independence can be devastating.

The new agents that block the endothelial growth factors that stimulate new vessel growth are, at present:

- Macugen (pegaptanib sodium)
- Lucentis (ranibizumab)
- Avastin (bezacizumab).

The third agent, Avastin, which has been found in pilot studies to have similar effects to Lucentis, is licensed for the treatment of bowel cancer. It is currently not licensed for the treatment of ocular disease.

LOCATION FOR CARRYING OUT THE PROCEDURE
The procedure may be carried out in an operating theatre or in a dedicated room. Within this clinic setting there are minimum

criteria, which have been outlined by the Royal College of Ophthalmologists' Intravitreal Injection Procedure (2006):

- Indications are a dedicated clean room as defined by local infection control teams, not used for infective procedures and free from interruptions.
- Rooms must have a washable floor and non-porous, non-particulate ceiling.
- There must be good illumination and an indirect ophthalmoscope is an advantage.
- Adequate hand-washing facilities must be available.
- The person doing the injecting must wash his or her hands and sterile gloves should be used.

CARRYING OUT THE PROCEDURE

A full explanation of the procedure must be given to the patient, which should include the following:

- The type of macular degeneration that the patient has
- The importance of the treatment
- What if any other treatment options may be available
- The importance of the intravitreal procedure and follow-up care
- What the patient is to expect during the procedure and any adverse reactions to observe for
- As part of a course of therapy, the treatment must be explained, the need for follow-up stressed and, if possible, an indication of the frequency and length of the course of treatment
- Consent for the procedure and additional investigations such as fundus fluorescein angiography (FFA) will be required; this usually covers the full course of treatment.

PROCEDURE AND PREPARATION FOR ADMINISTRATION OF INTRAVITREAL THERAPY

A number of investigations are carried out before the patient is assessed for the intravitreal injection procedure; these may include:

- LogMAR visual acuity testing (see Chapter 57, Visual acuity testing)
- Optical coherence tomography (OCT)
- FFA
- Pupillary dilatation with mydriatic drops such as tropicamide 1% to aid fundus examination by the doctor.

Equipment needed
- Drape
- Eyelid speculum
- Surgical gloves
- Micro-forceps
- Cotton buds
- Calliper measure
- Povidone–iodine for cleaning
- 27–30G needle
- Local anaesthetic drops such as oxybuprocaine (Minims oxybuprocaine) 0.4%
- Antibiotic drops, for example, chloramphenicol or ofloxacin to be used after the procedure.

Procedure
- Application of local anaesthetic drops before the procedure.
- Hand washing and application of sterile gloves.
- Instil 5% povidone iodine and allow a minimum of 3 min before starting the procedure.
- Cleansing of the skin with particular attention to eyelid margin with iodine is important before application of the sterile drape.
- Insert the eyelid speculum.
- Further application of topical anaesthetic may be applied, plus supplemental subconjunctival anaesthetic may be considered in some patients.
- The patient should be instructed to look away from the site of the injection; usually the inferotemporal quadrant is chosen.
- Marking of the injection site is important. Using a gauge set for the correct distance (rather than measuring the eye),

30

measure from the area of the limbus. If the patient is pseudo-phakic, 3.5 mm is the required distance. In phakic patients 4.0 mm is indicated.

- Gloves may be changed at this stage and preparation for the injection made, depending upon the drug to be used; this may or may not be via a pre-loaded syringe. Any air must be expelled before injection.
- Forceps or a sterile cotton bud may be used to steady the eye.
- The needle should be inserted at an angle towards the globe, avoiding contact with the posterior lens.
- The appropriate volume, usually between 0.05 and 0.1 mL (depending upon the preparation – see manufacturer's recommendations), should be administered slowly.
- The needle is then removed slowly and a sterile bud applied to prevent reflux of any medication.
- All sharps – needle, syringes, bottles – should be disposed of safely and the area of injection marked in the patient notes.
- Apply one to two drops of antibiotics to the treated eye immediately and then instruct the patient to use the antibiotic drops three times daily for a further 3 days.
- Check that the patient is able to see objects – hand motions – immediately after injection and look to see if the retinal artery is perfused.

POST-INJECTION PROCEDURES

Patients must be further instructed about the use of the antibiotic therapy; hand washing should be stressed.

Patients should also be asked to report any signs or symptoms relating to:

- Eye pain or discomfort
- Increased redness
- Additional blurring of vision
- Loss of vision.

These signs and symptoms could indicate endophthalmitis, which would need to be treated without delay.

Foreign body sensation can be noted for a 24- to 48-hour period or minimal floaters; both of these symptoms, although troublesome, should resolve spontaneously, the floaters after a few days to 1 week.

REFERENCE
The Royal College of Ophthalmologists (2006). *Intravitreal Injection Procedure Guideline*. London: RCOphth.

Photodynamic therapy

Clinical practice for preparation and infusion of verteporfin

Note that sterile technique must be maintained throughout all procedures.

	Action	Rationale
1.	Explain and discuss the procedure with the patient	To ensure that the patient understands and consents to treatment
2.	Assemble all equipment required	To minimise interruptions once the procedure has started
	Verteporfin reconstitution	
3.	Withdraw 7 mL sterile water into a 10 mL syringe using standard syringe needle and inject it into the 15 mg vial of verteporfin	Volume required to reconstitute drug to 2 mg/mL
4.	Gently agitate the vial until fully mixed and set aside leaving the needle and syringe *in situ*	To dissolve the verteporfin powder without causing the powder to 'froth'
5.	Withdraw the calculated amount (according to patient's body surface area or BSA) of D5W into a 50 mL syringe using standard syringe needle	
6.	Pull back the plunger to the 30 mL line	To leave space for adding verteporfin into the syringe
7.	Withdraw calculated amount (according to patient's BSA) of verteporfin into the attached syringe. Remove it from the vial and inject it into the 50 mL syringe	Total volume of fluid is now 30 mL ready for controlled infusion
	Using Y connector	
8.	In sequence, connect the 50 mL syringe containing verteporfin and D5W to the Y-shaped end of the infusion pump extension, a 1.2-μm filter, and then the infusion line	To prevent spillage from the syringe

Action	Rationale
Using standard infusion tubing	
9. In sequence, connect the 1.2-µm filter directly onto the end of the 50 mL syringe containing verteporfin and D5W, then the infusion line to the other side of the filter	
10. Depress the plunger of the 50 mL syringe until there is evidence of fluid right to the end of the infusion line	Correct priming of filter and tubing
11. Withdraw 10 mL D5W from infusion bag into two separate 5 mL syringes	In preparation for checking patency and flushing infusion set
12. Insert intravenous cannula into the patient's vein (antecubital fossa) as per local policy and flush with 5 mL D5W	To gain venous access and check patency
13. Load the prepared syringe into the infusion pump	
14. Set the pump to deliver 30 mL in 10 min (3 mL/min or 180 mL/h)	
15. Connect prepared infusion line to the cannula	
16. Set a separate timer for 15 min and synchronise the start of this timer simultaneously with the start of the infusion pump	To ensure laser is applied exactly 15 min after start of the infusion
17. After infusion, flush the filter and tubing with 5 mL D5W manually over a 60-second period	To ensure that the full dose of verteporfin is delivered
18. Remove cannula and cover site with sterile dressing	To ensure patient comfort and prevent cross-infection
19. Instil local anaesthetic into the eye to be treated	To anaesthetise eye before the insertion of contact lens
20. 15 min after initiation of infusion proceed with laser treatment	Optimum time for enhanced selectivity of verteporfin in PDT therapy

Section 7

Neuro-ophthalmology

Cranial nerve III palsy

DEFINITION
Cranial Nerve (CN) III, the oculomotor nerve, is responsible for the innervation of all the extraocular muscles except superior oblique and lateral rectus. Reduced ability of CN III will result in a variety of visual symptoms, which generally speaking result in problems with diplopia when both eyes are open.

SIGNS AND SYMPTOMS
It is usually painless with a sudden onset; individuals usually notice a diplopia on a certain position of gaze. This is replicable every time that the patient looks in that direction.

The diplopia will disappear if one eye is closed and positions of gaze are duplicated. The affected eye eyelid may be droopy and the pupil may or may not be dilated.

Dependent on the cause, the patient may also complain of other seemingly unrelated physical symptoms, such as lethargy, as the day goes.

DIAGNOSIS
Diagnosis can be first elicited by careful history taking from the patient. Details should be particularly taken to ascertain initial onset of signs or symptoms and whether or not painful (particularly on movement; Webb 2004).

Painful CN III palsy, with or without pupil involvement, must be referred to the neurosurgical team immediately because a cranial aneurysm must be excluded (Kunimoto et al. 2004). Further information is necessary to see whether the symptoms have taken a persistent and linear course and whether there have been any periods of remission. Such periods discount certain causative neurological disorders such as continuing raised intra-cranial pressure (ICP) and stroke.

Diagnosis can be confirmed on eliciting a symptomatic or sign response to 'follow my finger' ocular motility testing, with particular reference to pupil size. Full cranial nerve examination should be performed and recorded. Detailed orthoptic assessment is required as well as medical examination including blood pressure and blood glucose measurement. Kunimoto et al. (2004) suggest that all children under age 10 years be scanned. Pupil dysfunction results from loss of parasympathetic input and complete third nerve palsies, whether or not painful, should be assumed to result from compression of the nerve and neuroimaging be performed.

CAUSES

Causes are varied, with around 25 per cent idiopathic, but, in those involving the pupil, posterior communicating artery aneurysm, tumour, cavernous sinus mass, herpes zoster (check corresponding ear for shingles) and leukaemia are common.

In pupil-sparing CN III palsy, microvascular disease such as in diabetes, giant cell arteritis (GCA) or temporal arteritis are among the most common causes; both of the last two can be confirmed on history taking and blood tests.

Congenital CN III palsy is often caused by birth trauma and children may present with a CN III palsy after viral infection or immunisation, and is transient.

LIKELY PROGNOSIS, CARE AND TREATMENT

Prognosis depends heavily on the cause. Common approaches include regular orthoptic or other ophthalmic practitioner review to monitor regeneration of the nerve. Initially, occluding the affected eye may be the best way of dealing with the diplopia experienced by the patient. Prisms may help to improve the field of single vision; Fresnel prisms that stick on to spectacle lenses can be a good temporary solution and the prism can be changed as the diplopia changes. If diplopia persists and stabilises, a prism may be ground into spectacle lenses. The likelihood for the patient is that at 6 months after diagnosis the nerve should have regenerated and symptoms resolved. After 6 months, increased psychological support may assist the patient to come to terms with an altered visual ability that may be lifelong.

There is no pharmaceutical treatment or management option for a CN III palsy; however, if the cause is found to be undiagnosed or poorly controlled diabetes mellitus, control of this, through oral or insulin therapy, may lessen the time for nerve regeneration.

Once the diplopia has stabilised for at least 6 months, strabismus surgery can be done by repositioning the muscles to compensate. This is a risky strategy because the visual rehabilitative results can be poor. Furthermore, if the nerve were to regenerate after surgery, the effects would be over-compensated resulting in worsening diplopia for the patient.

Botulinum toxin injections may be used to weaken the overacting muscle to help achieve binocular vision.

Common risks to the patient include permanent diplopia. The condition may impact on patients' livelihoods and environmental abilities to cope. Simply put, patients could become unemployed or have difficulty in everyday tasks such as making a cup of tea or judging the distance of an oncoming car when crossing the road.

FOLLOW-UP CARE

In the intervening period between presentation to ophthalmology and the wait-and-see period for monitoring the condition, particular care should be provided to the patient with regard to the adjustment to life with visual impairment. Although the patient will not experience diplopia in all positions of gaze, the effects of the CN III palsy are still likely to alter lifestyle considerably.

This is the same for all age groups from students to elderly people. Referral to the appropriate agencies is advised, such as the local council's sensory impairment team/social work department, the local Department of Work and Pensions and, for students, the local education authority (LEA).

PATIENT EDUCATION

Patient education should, first and foremost, centre on what has happened and what is likely to happen. Although no certainties can be given at initial presentation or diagnosis, the patient's understanding of the palsy and its effects helps to gain patient compliance – such compliance minimising possible causative factors assists in nerve regeneration. Second, but just as important, compliance ensures that patients understand the condition and are likely to act to maintain a responsible attitude to treatment, monitoring the safety of themselves and others by heeding advice about activities such as smoking and driving.

REFERENCES

Kunimoto DY, Kanitkar KD, Makar MS (2004). *The Wills' Eye Manual, Office and Emergency Room Diagnosis and Treatment of Eye Disease*, 4th edn. Philadelphia: Lippincott, Williams & Wilkins.

Webb LA (2004). *Manual of Eye Emergencies: Diagnosis and management*, 2nd edn. London: Butterworth-Heinemann.

Cranial nerve IV palsy

33

DEFINITION

Cranial Nerve (CN) IV, the trochlear nerve, is responsible for the innervation of just the superior oblique (SO) muscle. The SO is the longest and thinnest of the extraocular muscles, and is responsible for the globe looking downwards, and also down and outwards and down and inwards together with downgaze. Reduced ability of CN IV will result in a variety of visual symptoms when the eyes are moved downwards.

SIGNS AND SYMPTOMS

The diplopia will disappear if one eye is closed and the position of gaze duplicated. Patients complain of the particular diplopia described above; occasionally they adopt a slight contralateral head tilt to the affected eye to compensate for it. Diplopia is increased if the head is tilted towards the affected side (Kunimoto et al. 2004). There is a risk to patient safety because the patient usually suffers from vertical diplopia, or diplopia with images horizontal to each other but remaining superior to the horizontal plane.

DIAGNOSIS

Diagnosis can first be elicited by careful history taking from the patient. Further information is needed to see whether the symptoms have taken a persistent and linear course and whether there have been any periods of remission. Old photographs are useful to see whether the head tilt is long standing or there is a history of recent trauma. Diagnosis can be confirmed on eliciting a symptomatic or signed response on 'follow my finger' ocular motility testing. Detailed orthoptic assessment is required as well as medical examination including blood pressure and blood glucose measurements (Kunimoto et al. 2004; Webb 2004). Eyes must be checked for facial asymmetry.

CAUSES
Congenital lesions are frequent and symptoms may not develop until well into adult life.

Vascular lesions of cranial nerve IV are common, but aneurysms and tumours less so. This is the most vulnerable nerve to trauma and, in older patients, microvascular causes are most common. Inflammatory or infiltrative processes such as the restriction caused by thyroid eye disease are also important causes of CN IV palsy.

LIKELY PROGNOSIS, CARE AND TREATMENT
These are as for CN III palsy.

A lack of recovery after 3–4 months should prompt neuroimaging with contrast to look for lesions within the base of the skull (American Academy of Ophthalmology 2006).

FOLLOW-UP CARE
This is as for CN III palsy.

PATIENT EDUCATION
This is as for CN III palsy.

REFERENCES
American Academy of Ophthalmology (2006). *Basic and Clinical Science Course. Neuro-ophthalmology*. San Francisco, CA: AAO.

Kunimoto DY, Kanitkar KD, Makar MS (2004). *The Wills' Eye Manual, Office and Emergency Room Diagnosis and Treatment of Eye Disease*, 4th edn. Philadelphia: Lippincott, Williams & Wilkins.

Webb LA (2004). *Manual of Eye Emergencies: Diagnosis and management*, 2nd edn. London: Butterworth-Heinemann.

Cranial nerve VI palsy

DEFINITION

Cranial Nerve (CN) VI, the abducens, is a small nerve responsible for the innervation of the lateral rectus of both eyes (Snell and Lemp 1998).

SIGNS AND SYMPTOMS

This is usually a sudden onset associated with no other problems; individuals usually notice a diplopia on looking left or right, which can be replicated every time that the patient looks in that direction.

DIAGNOSIS

Diagnosis can be first elicited by careful history taking from the patient. Details should be particularly taken to ascertain initial onset of signs or symptoms and whether or not painful (particularly on movement; Webb 2004).

Further information is needed to see whether the symptoms have taken a persistent and linear course and whether there have been any periods of remission. Such periods of remission discount certain causative neurological disorders such as continuing raised ICP and stroke.

Diagnosis can be confirmed on eliciting a symptomatic or signed response on 'follow my finger' ocular motility testing, with particular reference to pupil size. Full cranial nerve examination should be performed and recorded. Detailed orthoptic assessment is required as well as medical examination including blood pressure and blood glucose measurement. Cranial CT or magnetic resonance imaging (MRI) is often required, particularly in patients aged under 40 (AAO 2006). Kunimoto et al. (2004) suggest that all children under age 10 years be scanned. Children often present after a viral illness and this has an excellent prognosis, but, if it is not resolving, neuroimaging should be performed to rule out intercranial lesions. CN VI palsy is also associated with leukaemia in children (AAO 2006).

A number of other conditions can mimic CN VI palsy and will therefore need specific investigation. These include myasthenia gravis (for which a Tensilon test is required), restriction caused by thyroid eye disease, medial orbital wall fracture causing restriction of muscle movement and myositis (Kanski 2007).

CAUSES
CN VI arises in the pons, close to the facial nerve. Damage to the this nerve within the brain stem may produce an associated facial palsy. Raised intercranial pressure may stretch the nerve, causing a bilateral palsy. Acoustic neuroma or meningioma in the cerebellopontine angle may involve CN VI and other nerves, causing, for example, deafness or facial palsy, an aneurysm, inflammation or a space-occupying lesion within the cavernous sinus and ischaemia from diabetes mellitus or hypertension (AAO 2006). The nerve is also vulnerable to injury. As with cranial nerves III and IV, microvascular causes associated with diabetes are one of the most common causes. Isolated nerve VI palsy in adults is usually benign.

Common alternative causes are neurological causes, such as stroke, and myogenic causes, such as myasthenia gravis.

LIKELY PROGNOSIS, CARE AND TREATMENT
These are as for CN III palsy.

FOLLOW-UP CARE
This is as for CN III palsy.

PATIENT EDUCATION
This is as for CN III palsy.

REFERENCES
American Academy of Ophthalmology (2006). *Basic and Clinical Science Course. Neuro-ophthalmology.* San Francisco, CA: AAO.

Kanski JJ (2007). *Clinical Ophthalmology*, 6th edn. Oxford: Butterworth-Heinemann.

Kunimoto DY, Kanitkar KD, Makar MS (2004). *The Wills' Eye Manual, Office and Emergency Room Diagnosis and Treatment of Eye Disease*, 4th edn. Philadelphia: Lippincott, Williams & Wilkins.

Snell R, Lemp M (1998). *Clinical Anatomy of the Eye*, 2nd edn. Oxford: Blackwell Science.

Webb LA (2004). *Manual of Eye Emergencies: Diagnosis and management*, 2nd edn. London: Butterworth-Heinemann.

34

... ...

Assessing pupil reactions

The three pupil reactions are;

1. The direct response: light is shone on to the pupil and it constricts.
2. The consensual response: light is shone on to one pupil and the other constricts.
3. The near response: when the eyes focus on a near object, both pupils constrict.

EXAMINING THE PUPILS

To examine the pupil the light should be dim and preferably directed on to the face from below, so that both pupils are seen simultaneously. Size should be measured with a millimetre rule (Kanski 2003). Anisocoria, a difference in pupillary size between the two eyes, may normally be found in 41% of people examined (Burde et al. 1992); however, anisocoria that varies with the degree of illumination is pathological (Kanski 2003).

Reaction to light should be brisk and full, and should be tested when the patient is fixating at distance to prevent constriction as a result of the near response.

TESTING FOR RELATIVE AFFERENT PUPILLARY DEFECT OR RAPD (MARCUS–GUNN PUPIL)

If the afferent pathway is completely compromised, no light impulse will reach the Edinger–Westphal nucleus and therefore no direct response is possible. The pupil will still show a consensual response if light is shone into the other eye because the efferent pathway is susceptible to impulses directed to it from the fellow eye. Complete afferent pupillary defects are uncommon

(a)

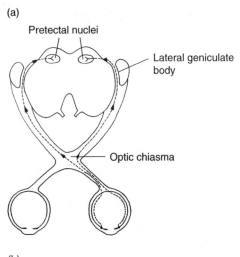

(b)

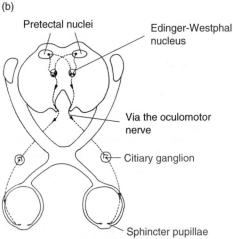

Figure 35.1 The pupillary light reflex – (a) the efferent pathway – (b) the pretecto oculomotor and efferent pathways. (From Needham 2006.)

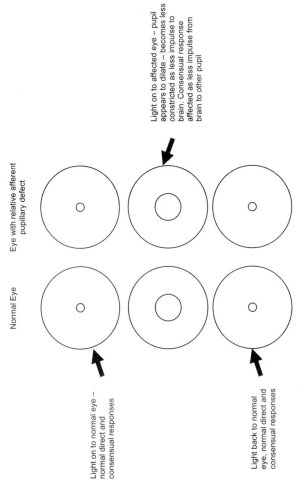

Figure 35.2 The 'swinging flashlight' test.

149

but RAPDs are a sensitive measure of optic nerve damage or disease.

The test for this is commonly known as the swinging flashlight test and should take place in a dimly lit room. Both pupils must be observed at once so complete darkness is unhelpful.

A bright light is shone on to the unaffected eye and the pupil's direct response and the consensual response of the other eye are noted. The light is swung to the affected eye and the pupil appears to dilate to a greater or lesser degree. Both pupils are larger at this phase of the test as a result of a lesser degree of constriction caused by a compromised afferent pathway of the affected eye and therefore a reduced signal down the efferent pathway. (In simplistic terms, if only 50% of the optic nerve is working on the affected eye, then only 50% of the 'signal' can reach the Edinger–Westphal nucleus and only 50% return down each of the efferent routes.)

As the light is swung back to the unaffected eye, its pupil constricts further and the pupil of the affected eye does the same (100% of the impulse reaching the Edinger–Westphal nucleus means 100% down each efferent pathway).

Although there are a number of ways of describing and classifying the degree of RAPD it is most often recorded according to an agreed taxonomy such as 'mild', moderate' or 'severe'.

REFERENCES

Burde RM, Savino PJ, Trobe JD (1992). *Clinical Decisions in Neuro-ophthalmology*, 2nd edn. St Louis, MO: Mosby.

Kanski JJ (2003). *Clinical Ophthalmology*, 5th edn. London: Butterworth-Heinemann.

Needham Y (2006). Visual and pupillary pathways and neuro-ophthalmology. In: Marsden J (ed.), *Ophthalmic Care*. Chichester: Wiley, 553–73.

Electroretinogram and electro-oculogram

DEFINITION

Electrophysiological testing of patients with retinal disease began in clinical departments in the late 1940s. Early intraretinal electrode studies enabled physiologists to tell which cells or cell layers gave rise to the various components of the electroretinogram (ERG) waveforms. Later, another diagnostic test called the electro-oculogram (EOG) was introduced. The ERG is a test used internationally to assess the status of the retina in eye diseases. The most recent advance in ERG technology is the multifocal pattern ERG, which is analysed and mapped by computer. It allows a detailed assessment of the state of the macular area.

USES OF THE ERG

Variations of the ERG test can illustrate diseases such as retinitis pigmentosa, myotonic dystrophy, diabetic, serous and hypertensive retinopathies, rod and cone dystrophies, retinal atrophies, Creutzfeldt–Jakob disease and many others.

Most retinal disorders produce a reduced ERG to various degrees. Others, such as Leber's congenital amaurosis and total retinal detachment, result in a completely absent ERG. Electrophysiological tests are used to elicit retinal function in infants and children and others who are unable to communicate effectively.

THE ERG

The basic method of recording the electrical response, known as the global or full-field ERG, is to stimulate the eye with a bright light source such as a flash produced by a strobe lamp. The intense flash of light elicits a biphasic waveform recordable at the cornea. The two components that are most often measured are the a and the b waves. The a wave is the first large negative component, followed by the b wave, which is positive at the cornea and usually larger in amplitude.

The a wave reflects the general physiological health of the photoreceptors in the outer retina and the b wave reflects the health of the inner layers of the retina, including the bipolar cells and the Müller cells.

The ERG of a normal full-term infant looks similar to a mature ERG. The ERG attains peak amplitude in adolescence and slowly declines in amplitude throughout life (Weleber 1981). Implicit times slow gradually with ageing.

Infants aged up to about 2 years can usually be tested without sedation while the parent holds the child. After that, sedation or anaesthesia may be required until the child is old enough to appreciate the needs of the test and is able to cooperate.

Recording the ERG

The ERG can be recorded in several ways. The pupil is usually dilated, and there are a number of corneal ERG electrodes that are in common use; they rest on the cornea.

There are also several methods of stimulating the eye. A strobe light is sometimes used or arrays of light-emitting diodes (LEDs). Single or several flashes may be used.

Method of carrying out an ERG

For more information see http://webvision.med.utah.edu/ClinicalERG.html.

1. The patient is dark adapted for a set time of 30 min.
2. Electrodes are attached to the cornea using dim red illumination (so that the eye is not light stimulated).
3. The ERG is recorded using single dim blue and red flashes, and bright white flashes.
4. Moderately high background illumination is turned on for about 10 min and the ERG recorded using high-frequency (30 Hz) flicker and bright white flashes. Responses recorded in this way show the cone system by bleaching rods. The cones recover faster and can follow the fast flicker better than the rods.

Rod and cone problems

Most disorders of the retina are detected by a smaller than normal amplitude of electrical signal. Timing and amplitude of waves vary depending on whether or not the eye is light adapted and the brightness and colour of the light flash. These parameters allow separation of rod and cone activities in the retina.

Rods and cones differ in number, colour sensitivity, the amount of light required to 'activate' them and recovery time. As a result of the massive preponderance of rods, the ERG after a white flash is dominated by their response. By manipulating the amount and quality of stimulation, rod and cone activities can be separated.

Rods are more sensitive than cones but cones recover faster. Cones can follow a much faster flickering light than rods and this can be used to test their sensitivity.

ELECTRO-OCULOGRAM

A standing potential arises across the eye as a result of ion exchange over the retinal pigment epithelium (RPE), with positivity at the cornea. Effectively the eye has a positive pole at the cornea and a negative one at the RPE, as in a battery. The EOG measures this potential and the variations in it caused by eye movement. If this is plotted as a voltage change over time, the EOG can graphically characterise eye movements and nystagmus waveforms. The EOG can assess the functional integrity of the RPE's interaction with the photoreceptors via the amplitude change in voltage, which occurs when ambient lighting changes: a light rise and a dark trough.

Skin electrodes are attached near the lateral canthus and medial canthus of each eye. A ground electrode is attached, usually to either the forehead or the earlobe. The patient is light adapted – for example, in a well-illuminated room – and the eyes dilated. After the electrodes are attached, the procedure is explained and the patient practises several times while baseline data are recorded. The patient keeps the head still while moving the eyes between two red lights. The movement of the eyes produces a voltage swing of about 5 mV between the electrodes on each side of the eye, which is stored in the computer's memory.

When the patient is used to moving the eyes, the process takes place again in the dark. Roughly every minute a sample of eye movement is taken and the lights are then turned back on with the patient continuing to move the eyes periodically. The potential rises when the lights are turned back on, reaching a peak in 10 min. When the size of the 'light rise' (or 'peak') is compared with the 'dark trough', the relative size should be ≥2 : 1. A light : dark ratio of <1.7 is considered abnormal.

It is not necessary to use the EOG as well as the ERG in most retinal disorders. Retinal diseases producing an abnormal EOG will usually have an abnormal ERG that is the better test. The most common use of the EOG is to confirm Best's disease.

REFERENCES
Weleber RG (1981). The effect of age on human cone and rod ganzfeld electroretinograms. *Invest Ophthalmol Vis Sci* **20**:392–9.

Visual evoked potential

37

This is a test used to detect sight impairment or blindness in patients.

DEFINITION

A visual evoked potential (VEP) is a potential evoked by sensory stimulation of an individual's visual field. Commonly used visual stimuli are flashing lights or checkerboards on a video screen, which flicker between black on white and white on black (invert contrast). The term 'visual evoked potential' is used interchangeably with 'visually evoked potential'. It usually refers to responses recorded from the occipital cortex. Sometimes, the term 'visual evoked cortical potential' (VECP) is used to distinguish the VEP from retinal or subcortical potentials.

REASONS FOR USE

Using monocular stimulation and an array of electrodes over the occipital region, it is possible to distinguish optic nerve, chiasma and hemisphere anomalies.

VEPs are very useful in detecting blindness in patients who cannot communicate, such as babies. If repeated stimulation of the visual field causes no changes in EEG potentials, the person's brain is probably not receiving any signals from the eyes.

Other applications include the diagnosis of optic neuritis, which causes the signal to be delayed. Such a delay is also a classic finding in multiple sclerosis. It can also be used to diagnose photosensitive epilepsy.

VEPs are furthermore used in the investigation of basic functions of visual perception.

37

155

TESTING

Monocular and binocular testing can be carried out. Monocular VEP testing is imperative if chiasmal or hemisphere dysfunction is investigated. An electroretinogram (ERG) and VEP are often used together in one appointment session and, in this case, it may be easier to have binocular fixation although account must be taken of ocular deviation and eccentric fixation.

The results localise the site of visual pathway dysfunction, and can monitor change and offer an objective assessment of the vision level that the visual pathway could optimally support.

CARRYING OUT THE TEST

Electrodes are placed on the patient's head, which may feel rather odd. The patient needs a full explanation and continued reassurance. The electrodes are attached at the right and left occipital lobes, located in the back of the skull. The electrodes used are usually silver (Ag) or tin (Sn), hollow-shaped domes, which are attached using a conductive paste to the skin over the appropriate lobe. To get a good signal (usually the signal output ranges from $0\,\mu V$ to $10\,\mu V$) from the occipital lobe the correct attachment of the electrode(s) is vital.

The signal received at the occipital lobe originates in the eye and is transmitted along the visual pathway, first through the optic nerve, through the optic chiasma, where the left and right optic nerves 'cross-over', and then to the occipital lobe where the 'image' is formulated.

CONSIDERATIONS

This process may be a little uncomfortable for the patient and, as the room is darkened, may lead to the patients feeling disoriented when the test is being carried out. Time must be taken to explain the process and length of time involved. Should photosensitive epilepsy be a possible diagnosis support of the patient in the event of a fit must be considered and made available before the test.

As a result of the nature of the tests, the patient's vision may be distorted immediately after them. A patient may require a few minutes to enable the retina to recover from the flashing lights.

FURTHER INFORMATION
New England Eye Center: www.neec.com
Institute of Child Health: www.ich.ucl.ac.uk

37

Section 8

Pharmacology

Section 9

Pharmacology

Administration of eyedrops and ointment

Most of our sensory perception is related to vision and so it is vital that as much visual function as possible is preserved. Eye treatment is, therefore, an important part of patient care; it has received very little attention in the nursing literature.

MEDICATION

Eyedrops and ointments are governed by the same controls as other medications. The *Guidelines for the Administration of Medicines* (Nursing and Midwifery Council or NMC 2002: 4) offer clear guidance on the administration of medication and state that:

As a registered nurse or midwife, you are accountable for your actions and omissions. In administering any medication, or assisting or overseeing any self-administration of medication, you must exercise your professional judgment and apply your knowledge and skill in the given situation.

The Guidelines also state that nurses should understand the correct dosage, therapeutic effects, precautions, side effects and contraindications of the prescribed medication and outline the nurse's responsibility when recording and delegating drug administration (NMC 2002). The NMC Guidelines go on to state that:

In exercising your professional accountability in the best interests of your patients, you must know the therapeutic uses of the medicine to be administered, its normal dosage, side effects, precautions and contra-indications. (NMC 2002: 6) and

> . . . make a clear, accurate and immediate record of all medi-
> cine administered, intentionally withheld or refused by the
> patient, ensuring that any written entries and the signature
> are clear and legible; it is also your responsibility to ensure
> that a record is made when delegating the task of adminis-
> tering medicine. (NMC 2002: 7)

EYEDROPS AND OINTMENT

Eyedrops and ointment provide a convenient and effective
vehicle for delivery of medication to a specific site, allowing high
levels of drugs to be delivered to the eye without significant systemic absorption. This reduces the possibility of unwanted effects
and also the quantity of drug necessary for therapeutic action,
allowing drugs such as chloramphenicol to be used topically
where systemically it is known to have potentially serious effects
(BMA, RPSGB 2007).

Eyedrop and ointment administration

Eyedrops should be administered by allowing the medication to
fall in drops on to the conjunctival surface.

For any drug to be effective, there must be enough absorption
from the site of application to allow maintenance of effective
drug concentrations at the site of action. Topical ophthalmic
therapy is prescribed at a frequency to allow optimum concentration of drugs into the ocular tissues, so producing optimum
therapeutic effect. Changes to the regimen of drops or ointment,
say by omission, can reduce the effectiveness of therapy (Fechner
and Teichmann 1998).

Topical ophthalmic treatments are used to:

* treat existing conditions
* prevent or treat inflammation or infection
* promote comfort and prevent damage to ocular structures.

Before the instillation of eyedrops the general state of the eye
should be assessed and any negative changes, such as inflamma-

tion, discharge or alteration in vision, noted and appropriate advice obtained.

One drop instilled into the lower fornix is sufficient because the eye cannot cope with any more fluid; more would overflow into the fornix, down the cheek and exit the fornix via the naso-lacrimal drainage channels. Excessive systemic absorption may take place through the nasal mucosa (Pavan-Langston and Dunkel 1991).

Adverse systemic effects can be minimised by asking patients to close their eyes gently for about 1 min after the application of treatment. This prevents the drops flowing into the nasolacrimal system where it would be unavailable for absorption.

It is advisable to leave 5 min between drops to prevent wash-out and non-absorption of the therapeutic amount (Pavan-Langston and Dunkel 1991).

Ointment should also be instilled on to the conjunctiva for absorption. This can be done by holding the lower lid down gently, applying a thin stream of ointment to the lower fornix. Where patients find this method difficult, they may be advised to apply a 'blob' of ointment to the caruncle/area of the plica semilunaris. The ointment will tend to become more liquid as a result of body heat and spread to the conjunctiva via the globe and lower fornix.

Various authorities suggest anything between a 1 mm and a 1 cm ribbon of ointment as a correct dose. The dosage of ointment is much more difficult to measure, predict and control than a drop (although drops vary in size depending on the amount of pressure used to produce them and different drop bottles produce different sized drops), so any ointment instilled into the eye must be judged to be an effective dose.

38

All drops should be instilled before eye ointment has been applied, otherwise it will not be absorbed and the patient will not receive the prescribed dose of medication.

SIDE EFFECTS AND CAUTIONS
Most eyedrops are also drugs and should be taken and given with the same caution and care as any systemic medication. Ignorance of eye therapies and their interactions can have

the potential to cause harm both in terms of eyesight and systemically.

Patients can experience allergic reactions to ophthalmic treatments, especially when preservatives are present. Advice should be sought from the person prescribing on the course of action to take and the preservative-free options available for many ophthalmic treatments. Drops should not be stopped for any reason without consultation with this person, because many treatments for eye conditions such as glaucoma are taken for a lifetime and a patient can remain asymptomatic, so, if a patient is receiving treatment at an eye unit, the ophthalmic team should be contacted before changes are made to medications.

Many eyedrops are absorbed systemically and can cause side effects. Non-selective β blockers, for example, may cause breathlessness and dizziness. Any patient who experiences breathlessness should be monitored. Alternative treatments may be necessary and also interactions between systemic medications should be considered, such as the reinforcement that may be achieved if β blockers are used both systemically and topically (Marsden and Shaw 2002).

REFERENCES

British Medical Association, Royal Pharmaceutical Society of GB (2007). *British National Formulary* 52, March. London: BMA, RPSGB.

Fechner P, Teichmann K (1998). *Ocular Therapeutics*. Thorofare, NJ: Slack, Inc.

Marsden J, Shaw M (2002). Correct administration of topical eye treatments. *Nursing Stand* **17**(30):42–4.

Nursing and Midwifery Council (2002). *Guidelines for the Administration of Medicines*. London: NMC.

Pavan-Langston D, Dunkel E (1991). *Handbook of Drug Therapy and Ocular Side Effects of Systemic Drugs*. Boston, MA: Little, Brown & Co.

Eyedrops that dilate the pupil (mydriatics and cycloplegics)

ANATOMY AND PHYSIOLOGY

The iris has two muscles:

1. A sphincter muscle that runs in a circular mode around the pupil and is responsible for constriction
2. A dilator muscle that runs radially and dilates the pupil.

The sphincter muscle is controlled by parasympathetic fibres of the oculomotor nerve (CN III) and the dilator muscles by sympathetic fibres from the ophthalmic branch of the trigeminal nerve (CN V).

The pupil can be dilated by enhancing the action of the dilator muscle or blocking the action of the sphincter muscle.

Tropicamide, cyclopentolate and homatropine block the action of the sphincter muscle (parasympatholytics).

Phenylephrine enhances the action of the dilator muscle (sympathomimetic).

TROPICAMIDE 0.5% OR 1%

Tropicamide takes 20–40 min to dilate the pupil; it is short acting, relatively weak and wears off after 6 h. It is useful for fundal examination of the eye.

CYCLOPENTOLATE (MYDRILATE) 0.5% OR 1%

Cyclopentolate takes 30–60 min to dilate the pupil; it is stronger and longer lasting – 6–24 h – and used more as a treatment for ocular conditions such as iritis, where it is necessary to keep the pupil dilated.

Table 39.1 Single dose ophthalmic medications and their actions

Drug	Initial response (min)	Peak response (min)	Duration (h)	Uses
Tropicamide 0.5%, 1%	Mydriasis: 20–40 Cycloplegia: 30	30–60	Mydriasis: 6 Cycloplegia: 6	Fundal examination
Cyclopentolate 0.5%, 1%	As above	As above	6–24 Complete recovery from cycloplegic effect could take several days	Treatment for iritis, corneal problems, etc. Fundal examination in children
Homatropine 1%, 2%	As above	Mydriasis: 40–60 Cycloplegic: 30–60	1–3 days	As above
Phenylephrine 2.5%, 10%	Within 15	10–60	3–6 2.5%: 3 10%: 6	Full pupil dilatation
Atropine 1%	Mydriasis: 30 Cycloplegia: 120	120	2–3 days	Iritis Rubeotic glaucoma Injuries/children

Information taken from Martindale (2003).

HOMATROPINE 1% OR 2%

Homatropine takes 30–60 min to dilate and lasts for 1–3 days; it is used as a treatment for iritis, corneal abrasions, etc.

PHENYLEPHRINE 2.5% OR 10%

Phenylephrine takes about 20 min to dilate the pupil; it can last up to 10 h, so it is used only when the pupil must be fully dilated or tropicamide does not have a good effect.

It has a vasoconstricting effect that can be useful in the diagnosis of scleritis/episcleritis.

Phenylephrine should be used cautiously in patients who have heart disease or high blood pressure (only use 2.5%). Side effects can include cardiac arrhythmias, hypertension and coronary artery spasm.

GENERAL SIDE EFFECTS

These include transient stinging and raised intraocular pressure; allergic reactions are rare but can occur with cyclopentolate and homatropine.

CAUTION

Dilating eyedrops can cause an attack of acute glaucoma in certain patients, so they should be used with caution especially in patients with a history of glaucoma. This pertains to patients with narrow angle glaucoma, for which dilating the pupil may block the drainage angle and trabecular meshwork. It is good practice to check that the anterior chamber is deep before dilating patients' pupils.

FURTHER INFORMATION

British Medical Association and Royal Pharmaceutical Society of GB (2003). *British National Formulary* 48, March. London: BMA, RPSGB.

Martindale (2003). *The 'virtual' – pharmacy. Pharmacology and toxicology centre.* www.martindalecenter.com/Pharmacy_6_HuD.html (accessed 24 October 2007).

39

Eyedrops and health-care assistants

There is nothing under medicines legislation to prevent health-care assistants and others from administrating a non-parenteral medicine. This assumes, however, that what is involved is solely administration (as opposed to supply) of non-parenteral medicines within, for example, the course of a business of an NHS trust.

If health-care assistants and others are engaged in the administration of eyedrops, whoever employs them must take responsibility for their activities, training, etc. and, as a matter of good practice, must have guidelines in place relating to the administration of the medicine.

ADMINISTRATION OF A POM: SECTION 58(2)(B) OF THE MEDICINES ACT

- The situation whereby health-care assistants administer eyedrops that are prescription-only medicines (POMs) directly to the patient's eye is 'administration' for the purposes of the Medicines Act 1968, so Section 58(2)(b) of the Medicines Act 1968 applies.
- Section 58(2)(b) provides that 'no person shall administer (otherwise than to himself) any such medicine unless he is an appropriate practitioner or a person acting in accordance with the directions of an appropriate practitioner'. There are a number of exemptions from this provision set out in the Prescription Only Medicines (Human Use) Order 1997 (the POM Order).
- One such exemption is Article 9 of the POM Order, which exempts the administration of non-parenteral medicines from the restriction imposed by Section 58(2)(b).

- This means that the administration of eyedrops classified as POMs can be carried out by anyone – that person does not need to be an appropriate practitioner and nor does she or he need to be acting in accordance with the directions of an appropriate practitioner, for the administration to be lawful.

ADMINISTRATION OF P MEDICINES

- Health-care assistants may also administer eyedrops that are classified as a P (pharmacy only) medicine to patients as part of their work. There are no restrictions in the Medicines Act 1968 on who can administer a P medicine, so anyone can lawfully administer one to a patient.
- Amendments to medicines legislation would be required if:
  - health-care assistants were to hand out eyedrops to patients, who will then self-administer them
  - health-care assistants were required to administer parenteral medicines in the course of their work.
- In the situation described in the first point, handing out medicines amounts to 'supply in circumstances corresponding to a retail sale' to which Sections 52 and 58(2)(a) of the Medicines Act 1968 apply. Broadly, under Section 52, a POM or a P medicine may be sold or supplied only by or under the supervision of a pharmacist, from registered pharmacy premises. Under Section 58(2)(a), a POM may be sold or supplied only in accordance with a prescription given by an appropriate practitioner. Exemptions to the restrictions imposed by Section 52 are set out in the Medicines (Pharmacy and General Sale – Exemption) Order 1980, and exemptions to Section 58(2)(a) are set out in the POM Order.
- The situation in the second point is 'administration' and is governed by Section 58(2)(b) or an exemption.

Prescribing and supplying drugs

PRESCRIBING DRUGS

Following the recommendations of the Cumberlege Report (Department of Health and Social Security or DHSS 1986) and the first Crown Report (Department of Health or DH 1989), the Medicinal Products: Prescription by Nurses, etc. Act 1992 amended the Medicines Act 1968 to allow district nurses, health visitors or practice nurses with a district nurse or health visitor qualification to prescribe independently from a limited formulary.

In 2002 further amendments were made to NHS and pharmaceutical regulations to allow a second category of independent nurse prescribers to prescribe from an extended formulary (DH 2002). It also enabled another category, the supplementary nurse prescriber, who prescribes from clinical management plans (CMPs) that are drawn up by patients' clinicians. The CMP is agreed with the patient, and supplementary nurse prescribers manage the patient according to the CMP and specific medication.

However, in November 2005 the government announced its intention to extend the prescribing rights of nurses further to any licensed medication for any medical condition (except some controlled drugs) (DH 2005). This became effective on 1 May 2006. Independent prescribing has been opened to other health-care professionals and prescribers are now known as non-medical prescribers.

INDEPENDENT PRESCRIBING

Independent prescribing means that the prescriber takes responsibility for the clinical assessment of the patient, establishing a diagnosis and the clinical management required, as well as responsibility for prescribing where necessary and the appropriateness of any prescription. (DH 2004)

Nurse prescribers must have done the following:

- Have successfully completed the Independent and Supplementary Prescribing programme for nurses and be recorded as an Independent and Supplementary Prescriber on the Nursing and Midwifery Council (NMC) register.
- Have a prescribing component on their job description.
- Practise within their job description, trust and unit policies and specific competency guidelines.
- Practise within the NMC Code of Professional Conduct with specific regard to 6.3 – practising within level of competence (NMC 2004).
- Carry out annual audit of patient management and prescribing linked to annual personal performance review.

SUPPLYING DRUGS

In the past, group protocol arrangements were used to enable the supply or administration of drugs to patients in particular circumstances. This system was ratified by the second Crown Review (DH 1998) which set criteria for the correct drafting of group protocols.

In England, it became mandatory for all NHS and general practitioner services to follow this guidance in accordance with HSC 1998/051 (NHS Executive 1998) and Wales and Scotland produced their own guidance (National Assembly for Wales or NAW 2000; Scottish Executive or SE 2001). Although the Crown guidance was comprehensive, the legal basis for such a protocol has always been rather obscure. It appeared that, while group protocols drafted to Crown Guidance were good practice, their use may well have been illegal under the Medicines Act 1968.

Secondary legislation was introduced throughout the UK on 9 August 2000 (Statutory Instrument 2000a, 2000b, 2000c). As a result of the change, group protocols are now called patient group directions (PGDs).

PATIENT GROUP DIRECTIONS

PGDs constitute a legal framework that allows certain health-care professionals to supply and administer medicines to groups of patients who fit the criteria laid out in the PGD. So, a health-care professional could supply (for example, provide tablets or eye-drops) and/or administer a medicine (for example, give an injection of systemic or topical drugs) directly to a patient without the need for a prescription.

The legislation (Statutory Instrument 2000a) states that:

Patient Group Direction means – in connection with the supply of a prescription only medicine . . . a written direction relating to the supply and administration of a description or class of prescription only medicine . . . or a written direction relating to the administration of a description or class of prescription only medicine, and which in the case of either is signed by a doctor . . . and by a pharmacist; and relates to the supply and administration, or to administration, to persons generally (subject to any exclusions which may be set out in the Direction).

In slightly clearer terms:

. . . a written instruction for the sale, supply and/or administration of named medicines in an identified clinical situation. It applies to groups of patients who may not be individually identified before presenting for treatment. (National Prescribing Centre or NPC 2004: 20)

The patient will require examination by the clinician in order that the decision can be made that he or she fits into the criteria for a particular PGD.

The Royal College of Nursing (RCN 2004: 5) interprets the instructions for the use of PGDs as:

PGDs should only be used to supply and/or administer POMs to homogeneous patient groups where presenting characteristics and requirements are sufficiently consistent for them to be included in the PGD.

WHO CAN USE PGDS?

The list of health-care professionals who can use PGDs is expanding but does not include health-care assistants.

WRITING PGDS

The law (Statutory Instrument 2000a) requires that PGDs should be drawn up by a pharmacist and the doctor who works with the nurses using them. In practice, representatives of any professional groups who are expected to give medicines using the PGD would also be included in formulating it. It is also felt to be good practice to involve local drug and therapeutic/medicines management committees and similar advisory bodies with medicines expertise. The PGD must also be authorised by the organisation within which it is to be used. In the NHS this is likely to be an NHS trust or primary care organisation.

In England, when PGDs are developed locally, HSC 2000/026 (NHS Executive 2000) requires that a senior doctor and a senior pharmacist sign them off with authorisation from the appropriate health organisation – that is, the trust – and that all nurses using the directions are specifically named within the PGD and signed by them (other rules apply in Scotland and Wales – NAW 2000; SE 2001).

REVIEWING PGDS

A PGD must be formally reviewed and reauthorised every 2 years and the review date should be included in the PGD. After the review date the PGD is no longer valid. The PGD should be reviewed immediately if changes in practice or evidence for practice occur.

A set of competencies is in place that should be achieved by all those using PGDs (NPC 2004).

PATIENT-SPECIFIC DIRECTIONS

There are situations in which patients may benefit from having a medicine supplied and/or administered directly to them by a range of health-care professionals.

To enable this to happen, independent prescribers can give a documented patient-specific direction, which instructs another health-care professional to supply or administer a medicine to a specified patient.

A patient-specific direction is used once a patient has been assessed by an independent prescriber, who instructs another health-care professional, in writing, to supply or administer a medicine directly to that named patient or to several named patients (for example, all the patients on a clinic list). Patient-specific directions are a direct instruction and do not require an assessment of the patient by the health-care professional instructed to supply and/or administer it, unlike a PGD.

REFERENCES
Department of Health (1989). *Report of the Advisory Group on Nurse Prescribing* (*Crown Report*). London: DH.
Department of Health (1998). *Review on Prescribing Supply and Administration of Medicines*. Report on the supply and administration of medicines under group protocol arrangements (Crown Report part 2). London: DH.
Department of Health (2002). *Extending Independent Nurse Prescribing within the NHS in England*. London: DH.
Department of Health (2004). *Mechanisms for Nurse and Pharmacist Prescribing and Supply of Medicines*. London: DH.
Department of Health (2005). *Nurse and Pharmacist Prescribing Powers Extended* (press release). London: DH.
Department of Health and Social Security (1986). *Neighbourhood Nursing: A focus for care*. London: HMSO.
National Assembly for Wales (2000). Review of prescribing, supply and administration of medicines; sale, supply and administration of medicines by health professionals under patient group directions (PGDs). Cardiff: National Assembly for Wales.
National Prescribing Centre (2004). *Patient Group Directions: A practical guide and framework of competencies for all professionals using patient group directions*. London: NPC.
NHS Executive (1998). *Supply and administration of medicines under group protocols*, 1998/051. Leeds: NHSE.
NHS Executive (2000). *Patient Group Directions* [England Only]. HSC 2000/026. Leeds: NHSE.
Nursing and Midwifery Council (2004). *The NMC Code of Professional Conduct: Standards for conduct, performance and ethics*. London: NMC.
Royal College of Nursing (2004). *Patient Group Directions – Guidance and information for nurses*. London: RCN.

Scottish Executive, Health Department (2001). *Patient Group Directions*. NHS HDL 2001/7. Edinburgh: Scottish Executive.

Statutory Instrument (2000a). The Prescription Only Medicines (Human Use) Amendment Order 2000. Statutory Instrument no. 1917. London: The Stationery Office.

Statutory Instrument (2000b). The Medicines (Sale or Supply) (Miscellaneous Provisions) Amendment (no. 2) Regulations 2000. Statutory Instrument no. 1918. London: The Stationery Office.

Statutory Instrument (2000c). The Medicines (Pharmacy and General Sale Exemption) Amendment Order 2000. Statutory Instrument no. 1919. London: The Stationery Office.

Topical anaesthetics and the eye

42

Topical anaesthesia is used frequently in ophthalmology for a variety of procedures. The choice of anaesthetic will depend on the type of procedure and the intensity of anaesthesia required. Short-acting anaesthetics, such as proxymetacaine or oxybuprocaine, are more likely to be used for removal of foreign bodies, syringing tear ducts or intraocular pressure measurement, for example. Tetracaine and lidocaine are longer-acting anaesthetics and are therefore used in procedures such as cataract extraction or subconjunctival injection when sustained anaesthesia is required.

Table 42.1 summarises the onset and duration of topical anaesthetics commonly used in ophthalmology.

If more than one drop is used the anaesthetic effect can last up to 4 hours.

Side effects are minimal; Bartlett and Jaanus (2001), Lawrenson et al. (1998) and Shafi and Koay (1998) all agree that sensations of stinging or burning produced on instillation are less with proxymetacaine than with oxybuprocaine or amethocaine. This makes proxymetacaine a good choice of local anaesthetic for children. However, lidocaine, proxymetacaine and tetracaine should be avoided in pre-term neonates because of the immaturity of the metabolising enzyme system (BMA, RPSGB 2005).

Topical anaesthesia is generally safe to use and few patients react adversely after instillation. However, Bartlett and Jaanus (2001) advise caution in repeated administration of topical anaesthesia because it may significantly retard healing of corneal wounds and can actually cause keratitis. For this reason local anaesthetic eyedrops should be used only for diagnostic or

Table 42.1 Onset and duration of topical anaesthetics commonly used in ophthalmology

Drug	Initial response (s)	Duration (min)	Uses	Side effects	Action
Tetracaine (amethocaine) 0.5% and 1%	9–26	≥10–20 High affinity for melanin so depends on colour of iris	Anaesthetising the cornea and conjunctiva Subconjunctival injections Cataract extraction	Conjunctival irritation, punctate corneal damage, dermatitis	Blocks sensory nerve endings near site of application
Oxybuprocaine (Benoxinate) 0.4%	6–20	≥15	As above Foreign body removal Eye examination in a painful eye	Rare, limited conjunctival irritation	As above Bacteriostatic action
Lidocaine 4%	Anecdotal evidence suggests 1–2 min	≥30	As above Used with fluorescein to measure IOPs	Effects of anaesthetised eye, i.e. corneal damage	As above
Proxymetacaine 0.5%	20	≥15	As above Foreign body removal Mainly used in children because it stings less than oxybuprocaine Used with fluorescein to measure IOPs	Rare, limited conjunctival irritation	As above

IOP, intraocular pressure.
From Hopkins and Pearson (1998). See also www.home.intekom.com/pharm/smith-ne/

procedural purposes. Patients should never be sent away with local anaesthetic eyedrops.

There is no need to pad an eye just because a topical anaesthetic has been instilled because the duration of action is quite short. Most people who come to an eye unit have a topical anaesthetic for applanation tonometry with no ill effects reported.

REFERENCES

Bartlett JD, Jaanus SD (2001). *Clinical Ocular Pharmacology*, 4th edn. Oxford: Butterworth-Heinemann.

British Medical Association, Royal Pharmaceutical Society of GB (2005). *British National Formulary for Children*. London: BMA, RPSGB.

Hopkins G, Pearson R (1998). *O'Connor Davies' Ophthalmic Drugs*, 4th edn. Oxford: Butterworth-Heinemann.

Lawrenson JG, Edgar DF, Tanna GK, Gudgeon AC (1998). Comparison of the tolerability and efficacy of unit-dose, preservative-free topical ocular anaesthetics. *Ophthal Physiol Opt* **18**:393–400.

Shafi T, Koay P (1998). Randomised prospective masked study comparing patient comfort following the instillation of topical proxymetacaine and amethocaine. *Br J Ophthalmol* **82**:1285–7.

Section 9

Trauma

Eye irrigation

The initial treatment of any chemical eye injury involves copious irrigation to dilute the chemical and remove particulate matter. Irrigation should start immediately, using whatever source is available. Herr et al. (1991) found no difference in the efficacy of irrigation fluids and therefore, the irrigating fluid of choice is physiological or 0.9% saline, generally delivered via a giving set to provide a directable and controllable jet. Sterile water may be used as long as appropriate equipment is available to ensure a controllable, directable flow of fluid. A running tap may be used to irrigate the eye or, in the absence of a continuous supply of irrigating fluid, commercial eye-irrigating fluid (which is usually supplied in small quantities) may be used. Buffer solutions that neutralise both acid and alkaline chemicals are available in some areas but are expensive and therefore not widely used.

Other irrigation devices include the Morgan lens (see www.morganlens.com), an irrigating contact lens that is attached to a giving set to enable hands-free irrigation. Practitioner experience of this device is variable, with differing amounts of patient comfort and compliance and irrigation effectiveness. Eye wash and eye irrigation stations are commercially available and often mix tap water with air for a very 'soft' spray of water, which is tolerated well by the patient. These tend not to be available in accident and emergency departments because of the expense of initial instillation but are very effective.

A drop of topical anaesthetic should be instilled before irrigation to assist in patient compliance and minimise pain. This may need to be repeated during the irrigation. Although repeated instillation of topical anaesthetic is not generally recommended, to facilitate effective irrigation and subsequent examination of the patient's eye, repeated instillation may be necessary to relieve pain and is desirable. Some clinicians report using an irrigating solution that contains 2% lidocaine to facilitate pain-free irrigation.

IRRIGATION PROCEDURE

- Before and during the procedure the patient needs information, explanations and reassurance.
- A waterproof cape or cover can help to protect the patient's clothing from the irrigating fluid.
- The patient should sit upright with head supported and tilted to the affected side (unless an eye wash station is being used).
- Irrigating patients' eyes while they are lying down ensures only that they will get extremely wet and are less likely to be able to cooperate in the procedure, as they strive to prevent themselves from what may feel like 'drowning'.
- Contact lenses should be removed before irrigation.
- The eyelids should be held open, manually or using a speculum, and all aspects of the cornea and conjunctive irrigated, including the conjunctiva exposed by everting the upper lid.
- All particles of chemical matter should be removed, by wiping with a cotton-tipped applicator if necessary.
- Particles may lodge under the everted upper lid, in the upper fornix. A wet cotton-tipped applicator should be swept under the edge of the everted upper lid and up into the upper fornix.
- Double eversion of the lid should be attempted.

It is impossible to specify an exact time for irrigation or volume of fluid that should be used because this depends on the nature of the chemical and its physical state, as well as the patient's condition. Wagoner (1997) suggests that it is impossible to over-irrigate a chemically injured eye, and recommends irrigation for 15–30 min. At some point, however, irrigation must be stopped so that assessment, examination and treatment can commence.

The use of pH paper to check for adequate irrigation may be debated. In alkaline injury in particular, the chemical will leach out of the eye for a number of hours after injury, thus altering the pH of the tear film. Delay in therapy of a number of hours until the pH is back to normal (neutral = pH 7, the conjunctival sac normal pH is around 7.4 – Forrester et al. 1996) will delay healing and irrigation for this length of time is not practicable or desirable. There is little in the literature to suggest **when** the pH of the tear film should be tested but, unless a number of minutes are left to elapse without irrigation before testing, it is possible that the irrigation fluid is being tested instead and this may lead to inappropriate cessation of irrigation. If this time is allowed to elapse before testing the pH of the tear film with indicator paper and the pH then proves to be abnormal, the eye has had a long period without irrigation in which further damage may take place.

Ultimately, indicator paper is no substitute for prompt, adequate and thorough irrigation and the clinical decision-making capabilities of the nurse coupled with a strong knowledge base will ensure that the decision to stop irrigation is taken appropriately.

After irrigation, the patient's visual acuity should be checked to provide a baseline.

REFERENCES

Forrester J, Dick A, McMenamin P, Lee W (1996). *The Eye: Basic sciences in practice*. London: Saunders.

Herr RD, White GL Jr, Bernhisel K et al. (1991). Clinical comparisons of ocular irrigation fluids following chemical injury. *Am J Emerg Med* **9**:228–31.

Wagoner MD (1997). Chemical injuries of the eye: current concepts in pathophysiology and therapy. *Surv Ophthalmol* **41**:275–313.

Padding/patching the eye

Padding of the eye is undertaken for a number of reasons, and the reason dictates the way in which the eye is padded. Padding should be undertaken only when the reasons for it have been considered. Loss of the field of vision of one eye is disabling and reduces the person's stability and ability to function in the world. There should never be an occasion when a patient has both eyes padded at the same time. This is, ultimately, likely to do more harm than good because it is psychologically as well as completely physically disabling.

TREATMENT OF AMBLYOPIA

Patching is the most effective way to treat amblyopia (Ryder 2006). The aim is to achieve best possible vision in the amblyopic eye by occluding the better seeing eye. Patching may be full time or part time and is undertaken under the supervision of an orthoptist. The patch is most effective if applied to the face rather than any spectacles to avoid 'peeping', and a range of patches are available for this purpose. The eye should remain closed beneath the patch to avoid abrasion of the cornea from the inside of the patch, or the irritation of lashes catching on the patch as the eye is opened.

PADDING THE EYE AFTER SURGERY

Eyepads may be applied after surgery both for comfort and to protect the eye. Where surgery has taken place under retrobulbar or peribulbar anaesthesia and there is disturbance of ocular movement and sensation as a result of the type of anaesthesia, some form of protection is required to protect the eye, and specifically the cornea, if lid closure is not complete. Although the eye must be closed beneath the pad, care must be taken that no pressure is applied to the globe.

There is no reason for eyepads to be used after cataract surgery under topical or sub-Tenon's capsule anaesthesia, although often a clear plastic shield is provided for use at night, to protect the operated eye.

Pressure patching may be required to control blood loss or swelling after other types of, in particular, oculoplastic surgery and the surgeon will prescribe this. Patients will need a significant amount of education about the pad and the limitations that it imposes on them (such as the inability to drive) and what signs and symptoms should prompt them to seek ophthalmological advice.

PADDING IN CORNEAL ABRASION
Padding the eye used to be part of the normal treatment for all patients with corneal abrasion in the belief that it aided healing and promoted comfort.

Padding in adults
A recent systematic review of padding in adults was undertaken in 2006 (Turner and Rabiu 2006). They considered 11 trials dealing with over 1000 patients. They concluded that treating simple abrasions with a patch does not improve healing rates or relieve pain. They did, however, find that those without patches received more therapy, such as topical antibiotics, ointment and cycloplegia, and other treatment, that complicated their conclusions.

None of the trials appeared to have focused on the size of abrasion and the reviewers suggest that further research be focused on large abrasions (which they define as >10 mm^2 – a circular abrasion of 3.6 mm diameter, for example)

This finding does tend to suggest that pads should not be used in the treatment of adults with corneal abrasion. However, there are some other factors to take into account. Use of evidence is not just its blanket application, but also its application to individual patients.

A trial of padding that shows, over a large number of patients, that padding makes no difference *overall* must have a number of patients whose condition is improved by padding – as well as a number whose condition is made worse. If all patients are padded, as used to happen in practice, those patients whose condition is made worse by padding are disadvantaged. If no patient is padded, those who might have benefited from padding are disadvantaged.

The extreme pain caused by corneal abrasion strongly suggests that the role of the clinician should be to try to ascertain which of those patients might be helped by padding.

Clinical experience suggests that many patients with large abrasions feel better with the eye closed, and padding helps to achieve this. The role of the clinician is therefore to find out from the patient whether keeping the eye closed helps, and then to inform the patient of the following:

- It might be worth trying an eyepad.
- We know that padding the eye does not affect healing.
- The pad is solely for comfort reasons so:
  - if it helps, it can be kept on
  - if it does not, or it makes things worse, it should be removed and any antibiotic therapy commenced.

In this way, evidence is applied judiciously and patients with abrasions receive optimum care for their individual circumstances.

Padding in children

Michael et al. (2002) undertook a randomised clinical trial of padding corneal abrasion in children, considering abrasion size and activities of daily living. They found at follow-up (20–24 h) that 85% of patients had 95% or more healing, and there was no significant difference between the padded and the non-padded group, even when adjusted for abrasion size. There was no difference in the amount of pain medication doses required. The only difference found was that the 'difficulty walking score', a measurement of a daily living activity, was worse in the group of children who had been padded.

This suggests that children heal very quickly and padding an abrasion in a child does little other than making them less able to undertake normal activities. Although the same arguments apply in that some children may benefit from padding, the very small possibility of a child developing amblyopia while padded, as well as the disorientation that padding produces, for which children are less likely to be able to compensate than adults, lead to the conclusion that padding for abrasion in children is neither effective nor appropriate.

REFERENCES

Michael JG, Hug D, Dowd MD (2002). Management of corneal abrasion in children: A randomized clinical trial. *Ann Emerg Med* **40**: 67–72.

Ryder A (2006). The orbit and extraocular muscles. In: Marsden J (ed.), *Ophthalmic Care*. Chichester: Wiley, 510–52.

Turner A, Rabiu M (2006). Patching for corneal abrasion. *Cochrane Database System Rev* Issue 2: Art. no. CD004764.

Foreign body removal and treatment

Examination of the eye will often reveal the presence of superficial foreign bodies, which must be removed.

CONJUNCTIVAL FOREIGN BODIES

Conjunctival foreign bodies are often easily removed (after instillation of a topical anaesthetic drop) with a dampened, cotton-tipped applicator. (All such implements touching the eye should be dampened with, for example, what is left in the Minims after instillation of topical anaesthetic, to avoid epithelial cells being removed inadvertently.)

Those that are not easily wiped off the globe should be removed using the same technique as for corneal foreign bodies, considering, beforehand, the depth of the foreign body.

If there is substantial staining on the conjunctiva, antibiotic ointment should be prescribed/supplied for comfort and prophylaxis against infection until the eye feels back to normal, indicating that the epithelium has healed.

SUBTARSAL FOREIGN BODIES (Figure 45.1)

Lid eversion (see Chapter 9, Lid eversion) should be an integral part of every eye examination. It can be done without anaesthetic drops. If a foreign body is noted resting on the conjunctiva lining the upper lid, on lid eversion it may be wiped off using the moistened, cotton-tipped swab used to evert the lid.

There is no need to use topical anaesthesia when removing subtarsal foreign bodies unless severe pain prevents lid eversion:

- It is unlikely that topical anaesthetic will have been instilled for routine examination and instillation, and re-eversion of the

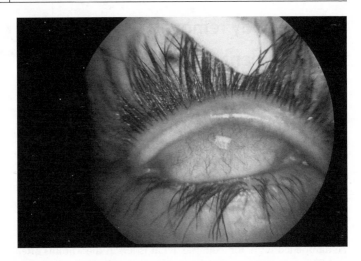

Figure 45.1 Subtarsal foreign body.

lid to remove the foreign body then lengthens the procedure and subjects the patient to two episodes of lid eversion that can be uncomfortable.

• Wiping a foreign body off the lid can be achieved very quickly, with minimum discomfort.

The patient will notice immediate relief from removal of the foreign body (Cheng et al. 1997).

If there is any corneal staining after removal of the foreign body, it is likely to be superficial and linear. Antibiotics should be prescribed for comfort (the greasiness of the ointment) and prophylaxis (against ingress of pathogens on to the cornea) either as a one-off dose, if there is minimal staining, or until the eye is feeling back to normal (and therefore the epithelium is healed).

CORNEAL FOREIGN BODIES (Figure 45.2)

Corneal foreign bodies are rarely removable by wiping. If they were superficial, it is likely that the action of the lid moving over the cornea would have removed them. They are, therefore, almost all impacted.

Before considering removal of a corneal foreign body, the clinician should be very confident about its depth.

The appearance of a superficial and deep foreign body may be similar on direct view and an oblique examination should always take place to check the depth within the cornea. Occasionally foreign bodies will perforate the cornea and protrude into the anterior chamber. No attempt should be made to remove these initially.

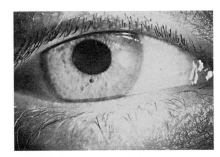

Figure 45.2 Corneal foreign body.

45

BOX 45.1 REMOVAL OF IMPACTED CORNEAL FOREIGN BODIES
There are two main ways that this can be undertaken and both involve the instillation of topical anaesthesia until the cornea is anaesthetised (limbal foreign bodies tend to need rather more time before removal is started to ensure a pain-free procedure). Both also involve a considerable explanation to the patient of his role in the procedure, which is generally to keep very still and look to where the clinician asks. The patient needs to know that a sharp implement is being used, that he or she will not feel any pain and that cooperation is vital in ensuring both foreign body removal and minimisation of any further trauma to the cornea:

1. Use the edge of a hypodermic needle (21 or 23 G) held tangentially to the cornea with the hand resting on the patient's cheek or nose. The needle may be mounted on a cotton-tipped applicator or syringe for easier manipulation.

   The metal is removed with the point or bevel of the needle or a combination of the two. After the foreign body has been removed, a rust ring often remains. This must be removed completely and is often easier after 24–48 h of treatment with antibiotic ointment.

2. A burr that is specifically designed for ophthalmic foreign body removal may be used to remove the initial foreign body, but more usually the rust ring. These are generally battery powered and possess either a burr or a brush tip (for example, the Alger Brush by Haag Streit).

There are advantages and disadvantages to both methods. The hypodermic needle method perhaps takes more skill and may sometimes take longer, but is single use and may be disposed of. The burr/brush is often felt to be easier to use when removing rust rings but does tend to leave a deeper defect in the cornea, which may be seen after complete healing as a small pit and, if central, can distort vision. This instrument also needs to be decontaminated and sterilised, and so a number of tips will be needed for use in any department. Clinicians tend to favour the tool with which they are most familiar.

Corneal foreign body removal needs to be carried out with extreme care. Although the cornea is tough, it is quite possible to penetrate it and, if the foreign body is 'dug' out too enthusiastically and the deeper layers of the cornea are damaged, a corneal scar will result. This might cause major visual problems if it involves the visual axis. Removal should always take place at a slit-lamp where the clinician has magnification and the patient's

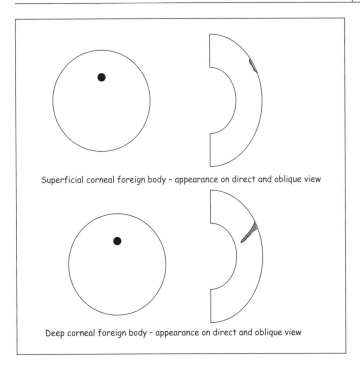

Superficial corneal foreign body – appearance on direct and oblique view

Deep corneal foreign body – appearance on direct and oblique view

Figure 45.3 It is important to assess the depth of the corneal foreign body. A similar appearance on direct viewing may change on an oblique slit view.

head is supported to help to prevent involuntary movement (Figure 45.3) (Marsden 1998).

The resulting epithelial defect should be treated with antibiotics (to prevent corneal infection), usually in ointment form (for comfort), although clinician experience suggests that, where the foreign body site is relatively deep, ointment tends to become trapped in the defect and, on re-examination, perhaps for removal of rust, the corneal tissue is rather oedematous in this area. Many clinicians therefore prefer to use an antibiotic drop in these circumstances.

Opportunities should always be taken for health education about eye protection.

REFERENCES

Cheng H, Burdon MA, Buckley SA, Moorman C (1997). *Emergency Ophthalmology*. London: BMJ Publishing Group.

Marsden J (1998). Care of patients with minor eye trauma. *Emerg Nurse* **6**(7):10–13.

Hyphaema

DEFINITION

Hyphaema is blood in the anterior chamber of the eye.

CAUSES, INCIDENCE AND RISK FACTORS

Hyphaema is usually caused by trauma to the eye, which may be a blunt or perforating injury. Severe inflammation of the iris, a blood vessel abnormality, or ocular tumours may occasionally cause bleeding into the anterior chamber as may interventions such as YAG (yttrium–aluminium–garnet) laser treatment.

A layer of blood in front of the iris may be noticed when the person remains upright for a while. A rise in intraocular pressure (IOP) may occur suddenly as a result of blockage of the trabecular meshwork by red blood cells.

SIGNS AND SYMPTOMS

- Bleeding within the front portion of the eye, between the cornea and the lens, in the anterior chamber – may be microscopic only, or visible with pen torch examination
- Eye pain
- Reduction in vision
- Light sensitivity
- Lacrimation.

EXAMINATION

- Eye examination
- IOP measurement (tonometry)
- Ultrasound testing to evaluate the remainder of the eye behind the front chamber.

TREATMENT

In some mild cases, no treatment is required and the blood is absorbed within a few days. It is advisable to rest, in an upright position, during this time to prevent further bleeding or complications.

Little and Aylward (1993) undertook a survey of ophthalmologists and found that patients were likely to be admitted to hospital for bed rest in most cases (even very minor hyphaema). The picture has changed massively since then, partly because of the reduction in beds on ophthalmic units and partly because of realisation that a re-bleed rarely occurs, the process and progress of resolution are the same whether the patient is sitting in hospital or at home, and patients are much happier at home than in hospital. Admission usually takes place only if there is a large rise in IOP, or a very large hyphaema and perhaps other injuries (Marsden 2006).

Children (and sometimes some adults) can usually be distracted by strategies such as reading, watching TV, and computer and other electronic games to keep them fairly immobile.

Patients should be advised to rest at home, with the head elevated at all times, including at night while sleeping, to allow blood cells to settle and absorb away from the visual axis. Red blood cells that are haemolysed while floating in the anterior chamber or settled on the corneal endothelium may stain the endothelium with haem pigment, which can affect vision. Central staining will cause visual disability and even deprivation amblyopia in a young child (Eagling and Roper-Hall 1986).

Advice should be given to avoid bending or lifting (raises the IOP) or sports (possibility of further injury) and not to return to work until instructed by the doctor. The patient will need to attend for review appointments to check progress and should perhaps avoid aspirin and ibuprofen because they may exacerbate any further bleeding.

Medical therapy in the form of eyedrops to decrease the inflammation or lower the IOP may be used if needed. Systemic therapy such as acetazolamide may be required if the IOP remains high.

Removal of the blood by an ophthalmologist may be necessary, especially if the IOP is severely increased or the blood is slow to reabsorb.

The patient will need to have a posterior segment examination, generally when the hyphaema has settled and the eye is less tender, to assess the integrity of other structures in the eye.

PROGNOSIS

The outcome depends on the extent of injury to the eye. Patients with sickle cell disease have a greater likelihood of ocular complications and must be monitored more carefully. Severe vision loss can occur.

COMPLICATIONS

- Recurrent bleeding
- Impaired vision through blood staining of the cornea
- Glaucoma.

PREVENTION

Many eye injuries can be prevented by wearing safety goggles or other protective eyewear. Always wear eye protection while playing sports such as racquetball or contact sports such as basketball.

46

REFERENCES

Eagling EM, Roper-Hall MJ (1986). *Eye Injuries: An illustrated guide*. London: Gower.

Little BC, Aylward GW (1993). The medical management of traumatic hyphaema: a survey of opinion amongst ophthalmologists in the UK. *J R Soc Med* **86**:458–9.

Marsden J (2006). *Ophthalmic Care*. Chichester: Wiley.

Ocular burns

47

Ocular burns may most commonly be divided into chemical, thermal and radiation injuries.

CHEMICAL INJURY

- The degree of injury is dependent on the type of substance involved, but, most importantly, on the length of contact time.
- Patients with chemical injury need immediate irrigation in order to minimise their injury (see Chapter 43, Eye irrigation).
- If the chemical injury is recent (3–4 h) the patient should be triaged RED – immediate (Mackway-Jones et al. 2005).
- All assessment, including visual acuity, should be delayed until irrigation has taken place.

Alkali injury

Alkaline chemicals include calcium hydroxide (lime, found in plaster, mortar, cement and concrete), sodium or potassium hydroxide, which are used as cleaning agents (for example, drain cleaner), ammonia, which again is used as a cleaning agent, and ammonium hydroxide, which is found in fertiliser. Alkalis penetrate rapidly through the cornea, combining with cell membrane lipids and resulting in cell disruption and tissue softening. A rapid rise in the pH in the anterior chamber may cause damage to the intraocular structures. Damage to vascular channels leads to ischaemia (Wagoner 1997).

Acid injury

Acids are less penetrating, precipitating tissue proteins, and forming barriers against deeper penetration and localising damage to the point of contact. Most acids are used in dilute form; however, given sufficient concentration, acids may cause severe ocular injury.

Thermal and/or contusion injuries caused by the temperature or pressure of the chemical may be superimposed on the chemical injury.

Sequelae of ophthalmic chemical injury

Minor chemical burns of the eye are likely to heal rapidly without scarring. More severe burns result in an acute inflammatory reaction. Corneal tissue is at risk of perforation as a result of the release of proteolytic enzymes from the white blood cells (Wagoner 1997). As the eye heals, formation of scar tissue may cause vascularisation and opacification of the cornea. Symblepharon may form and limit lid closure and eye movement. The lids may be damaged and this can result in trichiasis, entropion or ectropion, and cause problems with lid closure and exposure of the globe. Dry eyes often follow a chemical injury and are the result of damage to lacrimal ducts and secretory cells.

Appropriate treatment must commence as rapidly as possible, to minimise long-term problems and maximise visual potential.

Initial management

After irrigation, the patient's visual acuity should be checked to provide a baseline.

Cheng et al. (1997) suggest that patients with epithelial damage, including less than a third of the corneal epithelium or a similar area of conjunctival epithelium, may be treated in the same way as a patient with a corneal abrasion; however, the eye may look deceptively normal as a result of tissue blanching and ischaemia, which need urgent assessment and treatment – a totally white eye after chemical injury may be a sign of severe ischaemia with a poor prognosis for vision. Accurate assessment of the condition of the eye is therefore vital.

Ophthalmic management usually includes the following:

- **Topical steroids**: to reduce and control inflammation.
- **Topical antibiotics**: prophylactic use to prevent secondary infection.
- **Ointment**: keeping burned surfaces apart with a layer of ointment will stop aberrant healing (symblepharon) and ointment also enhances patient comfort.
- **Mydriatics**, such as cyclopentolate 1% to dilate the pupil, reduce pain caused by ciliary spasm and prevent adhesions between the iris and the lens (posterior synechiae) resulting from intraocular inflammation.
- Less often, **potassium ascorbate drops** or **systemic ascorbic acid**: after alkali injury, ascorbate levels become depressed. This substance is believed to be necessary for the synthesis of collagen. Although prescribed to assist healing, there is no evidence that these substances have any effect in humans (Mackway-Jones and Marsden 2003). Instillation of a weak acid into a damaged eye is extremely painful and therefore admission to hospital may be required
- **Rodding**: to prevent symblepharon. The technique involves using a glass rod and antibiotic ointment. The ointment is instilled into the eye and the rod is used, after instillation of topical anaesthetic, to spread the ointment over all surfaces of the conjunctiva, particularly in the upper and lower fornices, to keep the surfaces of conjunctiva apart and prevent the formation of adhesions.

47

Solvent burns

Injury caused by solvents such as petrol, perfume, alcohol and volatile cleaning fluids, although very painful initially, tend to cause only minor and transient injury. After injury, the patient often experiences acute and severe pain and 'stinging' in the eye, which may have settled somewhat at presentation. On examination, the eye is likely to be generally 'red' and punctate stains are seen on the cornea after instillation of fluorescein. Treatment of solvent injury is generally with antibiotic ointment to prevent infection and to aid comfort. Pupil dilatation may help if ciliary spasm is present. Reassurance should be given that this type of injury resolves very quickly and is not likely to have any permanent effects.

THERMAL BURNS

These usually involve damage to the lids (because the lids close as a protective reflex), although any other external eye structures may be injured. Superficial burns to the eye, such as those from hot sparks or ash, may be treated as abrasions. More severe burns may need similar management to chemical injury. Treatment of burns to lid skin is similar to that of thermal burns elsewhere on the body. Thermal burns involving the lids can heal aberrantly, with scarring and tethering of lid skin and conjunctiva, leading to lid closure and mobility problems, and oculoplastic surgeons should be involved at an early stage. The eye should not be padded if lid burns are present (Onofrey et al. 1998).

RADIATION BURNS

The most common radiation burns encountered in practice are caused by ultraviolet (UV) light. Causes of these are most commonly from welding ('welding flash' or 'arc eye') or the use of strong UV tanning lamps. The UV light is absorbed by the corneal epithelium and causes cell death. There is a latent period of between 6 and 12 hours before symptoms are noticed and this tends to depend on the amount of exposure.

The UV-damaged epithelial cells slough off exposing nerve fibres, causing pain that may be intense and be accompanied by photophobia, watering and lid erythema. Staining with fluorescein will reveal punctate epithelial erosions and treatment is as for corneal abrasion, with antibiotics as a prophylactic, lubricant for comfort, mydriasis if ciliary spasm is present and a pad (over one eye only) if it makes the eye more comfortable. Metal inert gas (MIG) welding can cause retinal burns because it produces high intensity white light (Marsden 2006).

REFERENCES
Cheng H, Burdon MA, Buckley SA, Moorman C (1997). *Emergency Ophthalmology*. London: BMJ Publishing Group.
Mackway-Jones K, Marsden J (2003). Ascorbate for alkali burns to the eye. *J Emerg Med* **20**:465–6.

Mackway-Jones K, Marsden J, Windle J (2005). *Emergency Triage*, 2nd edn. London: BMJ Publishing Group.

Marsden J (2006). The care of patients presenting with acute problems. In: Marsden J (ed.), *Ophthalmic Care*. Chichester: Wiley, 209–52.

Onofrey BE, Skorin L Jr, Holdeman NR (1998). *Ocular Therapeutics Handbook*. Philadelphia: Lippincott-Raven.

Wagoner MD (1997). Chemical injuries of the eye: current concepts in pathophysiology and therapy. *Surv Ophthalmol* **41**:275–313.

47

Sprayed chemicals and the eye

48

CS GAS

CS or 2-chlorobenzalmalononitrile is a substance that is used as a riot control agent and is suggested to be harmless by the groups who use it. CS was discovered by two Americans, Ben Carson and Roger Staughton, in 1928, the first letters of the scientists' surnames giving the name of the substance, 'CS'.

Around 15 different types of tear gas have been tested world-wide. CS has become the most popular because of its strong effect and lack of toxicity compared with other similar chemical agents. The effect of CS on a person will depend on whether it is packaged as a solution or an aerosol; the size of solution droplets and of the CS particulates after evaporation are factors that determine its effect on the human body.

CS Incapacitant Spray is used as a temporary incapacitant, to subdue attackers, or people who are violently aggressive, by many police forces. The chemical reacts with moisture on the skin and in the eyes, causing a burning sensation with pronounced lacrimation. Blepharospasm and conjunctival oedema may occur. When inhaled, the gas irritates the nose, mouth, upper airways and lungs. Profuse secretion is provoked. Contact stimulates secretion of large quantities of mucus and this, combined with the filtering mechanism in the upper respiratory tract, strains off the larger particles.

Locally, the gas causes rhinorrhoea, nasal congestion and irritation. If inhaled, particularly in a confined space, it can cause sore throat, coughing, bronchorrhoea, bronchospasm, in people with asthma, and pneumonia and even apnoea. It is particularly dangerous in people with pulmonary diseases. People who have had contact with CS sometimes develop allergic contact dermatitis (Sommer and Wilkinson 1999), even with blisters and

48

crusting (Karalliedde et al. 2000; Weir 2001). Studies show that most of the effects are relatively short term, but individuals notice some mild effects even after months (Karagama et al. 2003).

The CS spray used by some British police forces has five times as much CS as the spray used by American police forces (5% dissolved CS and 1% CS, respectively – Southward 2000).

The preferred treatment for ocular injury caused by CS gas is to blow dry air directly on to the eye, with an electric fan if available. This helps the dissolved CS gas to vaporise, and the irritation should disappear quickly. Rinsing the eye without having done this can further induce and prolong the severe burning sensation (Yih 1995). The casualty's facial skin and hair are best decontaminated by washing in cool water (Gray 1995).

The corneal epithelium usually remains intact and visual acuity quickly returns to normal. Minor disturbance, such as mild conjunctival injection and punctate fluorescein staining of the cornea, remains. Treatment with chloramphenicol or fucithalmic until the eye feels back to normal is suggested.

There have been reports of more major injury associated with discharge of tear gas at close range, including powder infiltration of conjunctiva, cornea and sclera, corneal oedema and vascularisation (Hoffman 1967), but modern methods of delivery may reduce this level of harm.

Particles on clothing may spread the chemical and lead to contamination of staff and other patients. If practicable, it is worth considering replacement clothing for the patient, the contaminated clothing being bagged for washing or placed in a well-ventilated area.

Other injuries should not be overlooked.

48

PEPPER SPRAY

Pepper spray (also known as OC gas or capsicum spray) is a chemical compound derived from the active ingredient in chilli peppers, or its synthetic equivalent, PAVA or Nonivamide, which irritates the eyes to cause tears and pain. It is used in riot control by a number of police forces in the UK. It is also used as an assault weapon. It causes immediate closure of the eyes and coughing. The length of the effects depends on the strength of the spray but the average full effect lasts around 30–45 min, with effects lasting for some hours (Department of Health 2004). Pepper spray is aimed specifically at the eyes and does not appear to have the same systemic effects as CS gas (Smith et al. 2004).

Vesaluoma et al. (2000) concluded that single exposure of the eye to OC is harmless, but repeated exposure can result in long-lasting changes in corneal sensitivity without a lasting decrease in visual acuity.

The spray used by the Sussex Police consists of a 0.3% solution of PAVA in 50% aqueous ethanol. It is dispensed from hand-held canisters (containing nitrogen as a propellant) as a coarse liquid stream; the spray pattern is stated to be directional and precise. The canisters contain 50 mL solution. The instructions are to aim directly at the individual's face, especially the eyes, using a half-second burst (still air) or 1 second burst (moving air), repeating if necessary. The maximum effective range is 2.5–5 m (8–15 feet) and officers are instructed not to use at a distance of under 1 m (3 feet) because of the risk of pressure injury to the eye.

Although there is no way of completely neutralising pepper spray, its effect can be minimised or stopped. Capsicum is not soluble in water, and even large volumes of water will have little to no effect. It is, however, soluble in fats and oils, and detergents can be used to wash it off the skin. Irrigation is useful to help flush the irritant and any particles from the eyes. A fan may be helpful in drying up the alcohol content, but even transient contact with alcohol causes pain and punctate epithelial erosions.

Treatment is based on the symptoms and injuries found, which are likely to be minor chemical irritation such as conjunctival or corneal epithelial loss.

It is worth bearing in mind that, if patients have been involved in riot situations, it has been reported that the electrical burst from TASERs can ignite the propellant in both CS gas and pepper spray, causing burns (Smith et al. 2004).

REFERENCES

Department of Health (2004). COT statement on the use of PAVA (Nonivamide) as an incapacitant spray. Available at:

www.advisorybodies.doh.gov.uk/cotnonfood/pava04.htm (accessed May 2007).

Gray PJ (1995). Treating CS gas injuries to the eye. *BMJ* **311**:871.

Hoffman DH (1967). Eye burns caused by tear gas. *Br J Ophthalmol* **51**:263–8.

Karagama YG, Newton JR, Newbegin CJR (2003). Short-term and long-term physical effects of exposure to CS spray. *J R Soc Med* **96A**:172–4.

Karalliedde L, Wheeler H, MacLehose R, Murray V (2000). Possible immediate and long-term health effects following exposure to chemical warfare agents. *Public Health* **114**:238–48.

Smith G, Macfarlane M, Crockett J (2004). *Comparison of CS and PAVA: Operational and toxicological aspects*. London: Home Office, Police Scientific Development Branch.

Sommer S, Wilkinson SM (1999). Exposure-pattern dermatitis due to CS gas. *Contact Dermat* **40**:46–7.

Southward RD (2000). CS incapacitant spray. *J Accid Emerg Med* **17**:76.

Vesaluoma M, Müller L, Gallar J et al. (2000). Effects of oleoresin capsicum pepper spray on human corneal morphology and sensitivity. *Invest Ophthalmol Vis Sci* **41**:2138–47.

Weir E (2001). The health impact of crowd-control agents. *Can Med Assoc J* **164**:1889–90.

Yih JP (1995). CS gas injury to the eye. *BMJ* **311**:276.

Surface ocular trauma: treatment

49

Conjunctival and corneal abrasions and corneal foreign bodies are one of the most common presentations to acute ophthalmic services. Once the decision has been made that damage to the eye is superficial, there are a number of decisions to be made about treatment.

Although surface ocular trauma is generally self-limiting, it is often intensely painful and limits the patient's mobility, occupation, sleep and ability to enjoy a normal life for a variable period of time. Treatment decisions will affect patient comfort and the patient's experience of trauma, and it is important that care be optimised for each patient.

The three main areas that need consideration are the prevention of infection, the treatment of pain and the optimisation of healing.

PREVENTION OF INFECTION

One of the eye's major innate defence mechanisms against pathogens is the integrity of the corneal epithelium. The eye normally has a population of commensal bacteria (diphtheroids, staphylococci, streptococci) that prevent colonisation with pathogenic bacteria (Forrester et al. 1996; Newell 1996). Disruption of the corneal epithelium allows penetration of the outer coat of the eye by these and any other opportunistic pathogens, which can result in infection of the cornea itself (infective keratitis) or of the interior structures of the eye (endophthalmitis), which can be catastrophic to ocular tissues and any prognosis for useful vision.

Any breach in the corneal epithelium therefore requires treatment with topical prophylactic antibiotic until the epithelium is

49

211

healed. Conjunctival epithelial loss is less likely to lead to ocular infection as a result of the nature of the specialised conjunctival immune system and because it is a structure in proximity to rather than part of the globe; however, antibiotic prophylaxis is generally given after conjunctival injury.

As antibiotics are for prophylaxis, the choice should be one with a broad spectrum of activity and, in practice, this is likely to mean either chloramphenicol or fusidic acid (Fucidin) preparations. Short courses of topical chloramphenicol do not appear to cause systemic side effects (Besamusca and Bastiensen 1986; Gardiner 1991). Chloramphenicol is available in both drop and ointment form and fusidic acid as viscous drops that become clear and liquid on hitting the tear film of the eye. Chloramphenicol is usually prescribed four times daily and fusidic acid twice daily, and this regimen should be continued until the epithelium is healed.

Often, a 5-day course is prescribed but the reasons for this are traditional rather than evidence based. It can be left to the patient's discretion to stop the antibiotic once any pain has resolved because, at this point, the epithelium has healed and the risk of infection has passed. The reason that a course of antibiotics is used in systemic infection is so that, when the infection becomes subclinical, pathogenic bacteria that are still around are not allowed to mutate and become resistant. In epithelial loss, antibiotics used are prophylactic rather than curative and, once the epithelium has healed, it can be left to do its job.

Practitioner experience suggests that ointment provides much more comfort, as a greasy surface between injured conjunctiva or cornea and lids. Chloramphenicol has an unpleasant taste and, as the lacrimal drainage system eventually drains down the back of the throat, chloramphenicol drops or ointment will be tasted for some while after instillation.

If perforation of the cornea is suspected or confirmed, a single drop of unpreserved, single-dose chloramphenicol (in Minim form) may be instilled before further assessment. Both preservatives and ointment are toxic to ocular tissues and should not be used.

DEALING WITH PAIN

Any breach in the corneal epithelium will cause a degree of discomfort or pain as the corneal nerves are damaged and exposed, and the extent of epithelial loss is likely to be related to the degree of pain experienced by the patient. Corneal pain is difficult to treat but a number of strategies can be used; an accurate assessment of the degree of pain is required and the pain experienced by the patient must be treated. Conjunctival trauma causes much less pain and foreign body sites, whether conjunctival or corneal, are usually described as being irritable rather than painful.

TOPICAL ANAESTHESIA

For examination purposes only and to obtain an accurate visual acuity assessment, topical anaesthesia may be used.

Repeated instillation will result in dose-related toxicity to the corneal epithelium and delay in healing as a result of inhibition of cell division (Fechner and Teichmann 1998). This means, in practice, that, if patients are given topical anaesthetic drops to take home, their pain will be relieved but the corneal epithelial loss will not recover and may get worse.

PUPIL DILATATION

A component of the pain experienced is likely to be caused by ciliary spasm where there is more than a very small area of corneal epithelial loss. This can be seen as the pupil of the affected eye reacts more slowly than that of the uninjured eye. Relief of the spasm, and therefore of a component of the pain, may be achieved through instillation of drops such as tropicamide 1% or cyclopentolate 1% to dilate the pupil. Of these, cyclopentolate 1% lasts the longer. The patient should be warned that these drops paralyse the ciliary muscle and therefore accommodation, and the patient's near vision, will be blurred because focusing is impossible. Atropine should never be used because it is completely irreversible and lasts from 10 to 14 days.

TOPICAL ANALGESIA

Prostaglandins play a major role in pain sensation and non-steroidal anti-inflammatory drugs (NSAIDs) are used systemically as analgesics to inhibit the enzyme cyclo-oxygenase and therefore decrease the synthesis of prostaglandins (Fechner and Teichmann 1998). Topical NSAIDs have been evaluated for us in corneal pain (Brahma et al. 1996) and found to be extremely useful. Their use does not appear to delay healing; no adverse effects have been found where the cornea is not otherwise compromised and the NSAID is used only for a short time. For patients with corneal pain, therefore, topical NSAIDs provide a significant degree of effective pain relief and are usually prescribed four times daily (Brahma et al. 1996; Fechner and Teichmann 1998; Rhee and Pyfer 1999).

Three NSAIDs are available as eyedrops: diclofenac sodium (Voltarol Ophtha) and flurbiprofen sodium (Ocufen) in single dose units, and ketorolac trometamol (Acular) as a 5 mL bottle that may be more cost-effective.

SYSTEMIC ANALGESIA

Use of topical analgesia should almost remove the need for systemic analgesia. Pain associated with other branches of the trigeminal nerve is notoriously difficult to treat. Practitioner experience suggests that many common analgesics provide little relief for corneal pain and other strategies, such as those discussed, have a rather better effect. If systemic analgesia is suggested, the analgesic that the patient normally takes is as likely to be effective as anything else, although NSAIDs have been reported to work well.

PADDING FOR CORNEAL ABRASION

To pad, or not to pad – that is the question (see Chapter 44, Padding/patching the eye). Padding should be an individualised decision made together with the patient and the symptoms, rather than a blanket policy.

If necessary, a double eye pad should always be used – one pad folded over the closed lids and the other on top of it. The whole is taped firmly to the face so that the patient cannot open the eye underneath the pad.

Medication (dilating drops, analgesia, antibiotics) should be instilled before patching and antibiotic ointment should be used because it will be present on the cornea for longer than drops. If comfortable, the pad should be left intact for 24 hours, then removed and instillation of medication started. If the pad is uncomfortable, it may be removed and medication started.

Pads should not be used in situations where the patient has to drive – driving with a pad on is likely to invalidate vehicle insurance and is, in any circumstance, very dangerous to the driver and other road users.

Patients should never have both eyes padded at once because this is extremely disorienting and disabling. If both eyes are affected, the worst should be padded and pads given for use at home for the other eye if necessary.

OPTIMISATION OF HEALING

Education is needed to persuade the patient of the importance of continuing to use prescribed medication to avoid corneal infection.

Decisions whether to review simple corneal abrasions depend very much on the individual clinician. It is useful to review large abrasions to ensure that healing is taking place and that there is no loose epithelium that needs débriding.

RECURRENT EROSION SYNDROME

Recurrent erosion syndrome is a distinct possibility for those patients who have an animal or vegetable cause for their corneal trauma (plant matter or fingernail, for example). The filaments that anchor the epithelium to Bowman's membrane may take even longer to heal and, until this happens, the epithelium is unstable and easily damaged. It is helpful to explain this to the patient and also that the time that they are most vulnerable to epithelial loss is at night because the epithelium sticks to the conjunctiva of the eyelid rather than to its basement membrane while the eye is relatively dry, overnight, and may be pulled off by the mechanical action of the lid opening on waking. This can be prevented until the epithelium is stable by using ointment at night before sleeping to keep the eye lubricated. 'Simple' ointment, or Lubri-Tears or Lacri-Lube (ointment base without drugs) should be used for a period of up to 3 months to prevent this happening (see also Chapter 22, Recurrent corneal erosion).

REFERENCES

Besamusca F, Bastiensen L (1986). Blood dyscrasias and topically applied chloramphenicol in ophthalmology. *Doc Ophthalmol* **64**:87–95.

Brahma AK, Shah S, Hillier VF et al. (1996). Topical analgesia for superficial corneal injuries. *J Accid Emerg Med* **13**:186–8.

Fechner PU, Teichmann KD (1998). *Ocular Therapeutics*. Thorofare, NJ: Slack.

Forrester J, Dick A, McMenamin P, Lee W (1996). *The Eye: Basic sciences in practice*. London: Saunders.

Gardiner F (1991). Chloramphenicol: a dangerous drug? *Acta Haematol* **85**:171–2.

Newell FW (1996). *Ophthalmology: Principles and concepts*, 8th edn. St Louis, MO: Mosby.

Rhee DJ, Pyfer MF, eds (1999). *The Wills' Eye Manual*, 3rd edn. Philadelphia: Lippincott, Williams & Wilkins.

49

Triage in the ophthalmic setting

In most acute settings, patients do not attend one by one, with plenty of time to assess and treat each person before the next arrives. It is essential to have a way of discriminating between those who present and to have a system in place to ensure that patients are seen in order of their clinical need, rather than the order in which they arrive.

There are many ways of achieving this and many systems in place in acute ophthalmic areas such as from simply 'urgent', 'soon' and 'delayed' categories to more complex methods.

When undertaken most effectively, triage involves a decision about clinical priority based on how the person presents rather than on the diagnosis. The triage encounter is not long enough to make a diagnosis, which may not be a good indication of clinical priority because, for example, of levels of pain (a perforating injury may be almost painless, but a large abrasion, much less urgent, very painful).

Effective clinical management of the patient and efficient departmental management depend on accurate allocation of the clinical priority in the triage encounter.

Whatever system is in place, it must be systematic, rigorous and auditable. It must also be seen to be fair in order that patients do not feel that there is discrimination involved in who is seen next.

One such method is that designed by the Manchester Triage Group (Mackway-Jones et al. 2005). This method is known as 'Emergency Triage' or, often, 'Manchester Triage' and was designed for general accident and emergency (A&E) departments. It has been adopted by most A&E departments in the UK and as a national triage system by a number of countries in

Table 50.1 Times allocated to areas of the national triage scale

Colour	Name	Target time (minutes)
Red	Immediate	0
Orange	Very urgent	10
Yellow	Urgent	60
Green	Standard	120
Blue	Non-urgent	240

Europe and further afield. It provides a standard to which ophthalmic acute or emergency settings must aspire. Manchester Triage uses a series of presentations and a limited number of signs and symptoms at each level of clinical priority. This ensures consistency between those who triage and transparency of the decision to allocate a clinical priority.

The method is reductive – the method starts with the most severe possibilities and works downwards. A patient must be allocated a higher triage category if a discriminator in that category cannot be ruled out. The system therefore defaults to a safe priority. From a general A&E department perspective, there are 52 presentations and the triage practitioner must decide which to use. From an ophthalmic perspective, there is only one commonly used presentation and that is 'eye problems' (Mackway-Jones et al. 2005). In the UK, the times allocated to areas of the national triage scale are as shown in Table 50.1.

The 'blue' target has since been modified, in line with UK government targets, which aim that all patients should be discharged from emergency care within 4 hours.

TELEPHONE TRIAGE
Telephone triage also has its difficulties because the patient is not visible, so many of the cues that experienced nurses take from the patient's appearance and behaviour are not available. The nurse may not even be able to gain information from the patient but may be talking to an intermediary such as a relative or neighbour or another health professional, all of whom may know the patient to a greater or lesser degree. This system can be modified

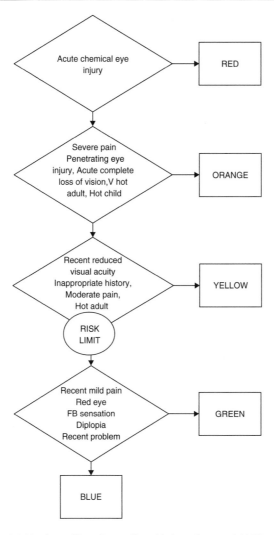

Figure 50.1 Manchester Triage System. (From Mackway-Jones et al. 2005.)

to allow consistent and auditable telephone triage, the discriminators being mapped to different decisions. These may be that the patient needs to be seen now or needs to be seen within a number of days, or perhaps that advice and self-care are all that is required in this episode. Advice may need to be supplied for care before arrival at the ophthalmic setting such as in the case of a patient phoning up to ask about a chemical injury. The ophthalmic nurse will advise that the patient make his or her way immediately to the eye unit – or a local A&E department if nearer to the patient – and in the meantime should wash the eye out with water or whatever is immediately available.

The conversation, including information from the caller and decisions made by the clinician, is recorded in detail.

Telephone triage, like triage, should be undertaken by experienced practitioners. The availability of any protocols and flowcharts does not remove the need for expert clinical knowledge. The decisions made in telephone triage arguably call for a higher level of skill and knowledge than when the patient is present and, certainly, the questioning skills of the practitioner must be very highly developed to gain the most useful information, quickly, from a worried caller.

Similar to triage, telephone triage works well when it is carried out correctly and less well when corners are cut, or aspects, such as pain, ignored. Systems must be auditable and this relies on good training of competent practitioners using their skills and knowledge and the tools available to them to the best effect.

REFERENCE
Mackway-Jones K, Marsden J, Windle J (2005). *Emergency Triage*, 2nd edn. London: BMJ Publishing Group.

Section 10

General topics

Peripheral venous cannulation is a practical skill that is universally employed throughout the world to obtain access for the administration of intravenous drugs (within ophthalmology often for the purpose of administration of diagnostic dyes such as fluorescein sodium and indocyanine green).

Peripheral venous cannulation is a practical skill that is underpinned by theoretical knowledge (keystone 1 of skills for health competence).

Teaching and learning strategies should be in place in order to assess competence to practice.

There are a number of considerations for those undertaking cannulation:

- Local policies and procedures
- Need for cannulation
- Informed consent
- Patient understanding
- Preparation for the procedure including the selection of the appropriate equipment
- Use of the appropriate site of insertion of the cannula
- Care planning for administration of the drug
- Documentation.

CONSIDERATIONS BEFORE THE CANNULATION PROCEDURE

Explain again all that you are doing to the patient! Check packaging and that all equipment and drugs are within date. Handwashing/cleansing before, during and after the activity will minimise and prevent infection.

TECHNIQUE

- Application of tourniquet to upper arm in order to distend the veins
- Select a suitable vein such as the antecubital vein
- Support the arm
- Estimate the size of the cannula needed
- Swab the chosen area
- Puncture the chosen vein with the cannula
- Remove the introducer
- Secure the cannula using an appropriate dressing such as Tegederm
- Check patency
- Dispose of all sharps appropriately in sharps bins
- Documentation.

COMPLICATIONS

- Failure
- Bleeding
- Extravasation of drugs into tissues.

Competence can be defined as the state of having the knowledge, judgement, skill, energy, experience and motivation required to respond adequately to the demands of one's professional responsibilities.

FURTHER READING

Campbell J (1997). Intravenous cannulation: Potential complications. *Prof Nurse* **12**(suppl):510–13.

Castledine G (1996). Nurses' role in peripheral venous cannulation. *Br J Nursing* **5**:1274.

Goodinson SM (1990). Good practice ensures minimum risk factors: complications of peripheral venous cannulation and infusion therapy. *Prof Nurse* **6**:175–7.

Roach MS (1992). *The Human Act of Caring*. Ottawa, Ontario: Canadian Hospital Association Press.

Royal College of Nursing (2005). *Competencies: An educational training competency framework for peripheral venous cannulation in children and young people*. London: RCN.

Scales K (2005). Vascular access, a guide to peripheral venous cannulation. *Nursing Stand* **19**(49):48–52.

Skills for Health Competence Database. CHS22: Perform intravenous cannulation. Available at: www.skillsforhealth.org.uk (accessed 3 August 2006).

Differential diagnosis of the red eye

	Conjunctivitis	Uveitis	Glaucoma	Corneal ulcers
Lids	? swollen Follicles, papillae if allergic	Normal	Normal	May be swollen
Conjunctiva	Injected	Injected	Injected	Injected
Cornea	? punctate staining	Normal, bright reaction	Very hazy	Opacity/stains with fluorescein
Anterior chamber	Deep	Deep	Shallow or flat	Deep
Iris	Normal	May look 'muddy'	May be difficult to see	Normal
Pupil	Normal	Slight miosis (compared with fellow) Sluggish	Fixed, oval, semi-dilated	Usually normal, may be slightly sluggish
Pain	Gritty	Deep pain in eye	Severe pain in and around eye and head	Gritty
Discharge	Pus/watery/ sticky in morning	May water	No	May water
Photophobia	If severe	Yes	No	Not usually
Systemically	? flu-like symptoms (URTI)	Well	Nausea Vomiting Severe abdominal pain Dehydration	Well

URTI, upper respiratory tract infection.
From Marsden (2006).

REFERENCE
Marsden J (2006). *Ophthalmic Care*. Chichester: Wiley.

Focimetry

A focimeter or lensmeter is an instrument that is used to measure the power of a lens. The sphere and cylinder (cyl) powers can be measured, the axis determined and the optical centre of the lens found. It is also possible to measure the bifocal addition on most lenses.

Before trying to measure any lenses with a focimeter, the eyepiece MUST be focused for you to see clearly. This is done by setting the machine to read plano (zero) and then adjusting the eyepiece so that the target and graticule markings in the focimeter are in focus. This means that the machine is now set for your personal refraction and any refractive error that the user has is neutralised.

The 'dot target' is the most common target seen down the focimeter viewing scope. A spherical lens will simply blur the dots, and adjusting the power dial will bring them into sharp focus. The power can now be read and noted. If there is cylinder power, the dots are blurred into lines, which can be brought into two foci. The most positive (or least negative) is the spherical power, and the difference between the two powers is the cyl power. The axis is the axis for the more negative power reading. Optician prescriptions normally record lens powers in minus cyl form, but this is a matter of choice and it is equally accurate to write it in the positive cyl format. The choice is up to your unit, but it is best to choose which format and to adhere to that for all measurements and recordings.

TECHNIQUE

Place the lens in the lensmeter, and adjust the dioptre scale until it shows a well-focused target (spherical lens) or until one meridian is clearly in focus (astigmatic lens); note the power and axis.

Refocus to obtain the second set of lines (at 90° to the first axis) and note the power and axis again. To calculate the sphero-cyl power in negative cyl form, select the more positive/less negative power as your sphere. Calculate the difference between the main powers (take the sphere power from the other), remembering the power signs – this is the cylinder power. The axis is the one found with the second power (not the one selected as the sphere).

Example

+1.00 × 90 and +3.00 × 180

The second power is the more positive and is therefore chosen as the sphere power. The difference between the powers is +1.00 − (+3.00) = −2.00

The axis is taken from the second, less positive power. In this case it is 90. Therefore the sphero-cyl power is +3.00/−2.00 × 9. The power of a lens can be written in three different ways:

1. +1.00 × 90/+2.00 × 180 – crossed cylinder form
2. +1.00 DS/+1.00 × 180 – plus cylinder form
3. +2.00 DS/−1.00 × 90 – minus cylinder form.

Transposition

The prescription for a lens can be written in several different forms. The two most commonly used forms are the PLUS CYL-INDER form and the MINUS CYLINDER form. For both forms the lens is effectively the same, but the written form looks very different.

To transpose from one form to the other:

- The cylinder POWER stays the same.
- The cylinder SIGN always changes.

The cylinder axis always changes by 90 (if <90 add 90, or if >90 subtract 90 to give an axis between 1 and 180 inclusive).

ADD the old sphere power and the old cyl power (always remembering the signs) to obtain the new sphere power.

FURTHER READING

Mayer S (2000). Refraction training manual. *J Commercial Eye Health* **13**(33):8.

Miller D (1991). *Optics and Refraction. A user friendly guide*, Vol 1. London: Gower Medical Publishing.

Heat treatment

There is little evidence available on the effectiveness of heat treatment for eye conditions, but it is widely used by clinicians and anecdotal evidence suggests that it has a value in certain conditions and circumstances.

A number of mechanisms appear to be relevant:

- Heat increases blood flow and tends to reduce inflammation and swelling. It may be perceived as soothing by the patient.
- Heat certainly aids the absorption of drugs through the skin (Kligman 1983; Hull 2002) and a similar mechanism may occur when the tissue concerned is conjunctiva. Scleral penetration may be facilitated if more of the drug is absorbed through the conjunctiva.
- Keeping the eye closed during heat treatment also aids drug absorption as the drug remains in contact with the eye for longer and is not washed away by tear movement.
- Application of heat is likely to soften secretions of the meibomian glands which may help in the treatment of blepharitis and styes or chalazia.

USES OF HEAT TREATMENT
Heat treatment is most often used in the following:

- The acute phase of anterior uveitis: during intensive dilatation (to aid with the absorption of medications such as mydriatics used to dilate the pupil and break down posterior synaechiae).
- The treatment of blepharitis: to soothe, facilitate lid cleaning and soften secretions.
- The treatment of styes and chalazia: to aid the absorption of topical antibiotic therapy, soften secretions and aid discharge.

RISKS

Burns to the eyelids are possible if the heat applied is excessive. Metallic implements should not be brought into contact with the lids.

WAYS OF APPLYING HEAT

Hot spoon bathing

A wooden or metallic spoon is heated in boiling water to allow heat absorption. It is removed from the water, dried and placed near to the eye. A metallic spoon radiates heat to the eye more effectively than a wooden implement but will also cause a more severe injury if placed on the lids.

A face sauna

A bowl of boiling water should be placed on a secure surface. The patient should sit comfortably and place the head over the steaming water. This may not be suitable for patients with respiratory disorders. Proprietary face saunas are also available.

A Thermos flask half-full with boiling water has the same effect but to a more localised area.

A hot glove

A non-sterile glove with no latex (to avoid latex sensitisation) can be filled with hot water from a tap, tied off at the wrist and placed over the closed lids, with or without a cover. The glove has an advantage of conforming to the eyelids and applying direct heat, so the water used may be cooler than other methods and there is less potential for injury. Glove manufacturers consulted have no objection to their products being used in this way.

REFERENCES

Hull W (2002) Heat-enhanced transdermal drug delivery: a survey paper. *J Appl Res Clin Exp Ther* **2**(2). Available at: http://jrnlappliedresearch.com/articles/Vol2Iss1/Hull.htm (accessed 23 October 2007).

Kligman AM (1983). A biological brief on percutaneous absorption. *Drug Dev Industr Pharm* **9**:521–60.

Infection control in ophthalmology

Hospital-acquired infection (HAI) is costly for both the patient and the carer, not only financially but also personally. In particular, there is public and professional concern about meticillin-resistant *Staphylococcus aureus* (MRSA) and *Clostridium difficile* infections.

It is well known that one of the most effective means of preventing infection is good hand hygiene and Lankford et al. (2003) found that role models play an important function in compliance with hand washing. They noted that, if senior staff did not wash their hands when juniors were present, the junior was likely to mimic that behaviour.

The World Health Organization (WHO) has developed guidelines on hand washing, including the importance of keeping hands well maintained and using moisturiser at the end of a shift (WHO 2005). In the UK, the 'clean your hands' campaign has reinforced this (see www.npsa.nhs.uk/cleanyourhands).

According to Jones (1998) immunosuppressed patients and those on steroids need to be protected from developing opportunistic infections and should be carefully monitored during the course of treatment.

EQUIPMENT AND INSTRUMENTS

Equipment such as slit-lamps and fields machines should be decontaminated between patients. Instruments should ideally be for single patient use; where they are not, appropriate de-contamination and sterilisation procedures must be followed (below). This is especially important in the prevention of the spread of Creutzfeldt–Jakob disease (CJD) (Department of Health or DH 2007).

Care of surgical instruments

This section draws on the work of Hawksworth (2006) for the Royal College of Ophthalmologists.

The theoretical risk of variant CJD (vCJD) transmission via surgical instruments has led to much closer scrutiny of the care and use of surgical instruments. Decontamination projects have been started in England to ensure that all NHS hospitals have access to services of an agreed standard.

A Scottish Action Plan has been introduced and this has been mirrored in Wales with all health service decontamination units being accredited to the EU medical device standard. The Council Directive 93/42/EEC of 14 June 1993, concerning medical devices, defines a 'medical device' as:

> ... any instrument, apparatus, appliance, material or other article, whether used alone or in combination, including the software necessary for its proper application intended by the manufacturer to be used for human beings for the purpose of:
>
> - diagnosis, prevention, monitoring, treatment or alleviation of disease,
> - diagnosis, monitoring, treatment, alleviation of or compensation for an injury or handicap,
> - investigation, replacement or modification of the anatomy or of a physiological process,
> - control of conception, and which does not achieve its principal intended action in or on the human body by pharmacological, immunological or metabolic means, but which may be assisted in its function by such means.

The Medicines and Healthcare products Regulatory Agency (MHRA) regulates medical devices in the UK under European legislation.

Ineffective decontamination can result in problems via four main pathways (Hawksworth 2006):

1. Foreign protein transfer, leading to risk of adverse reaction, or transmission of CJD in the case of prion protein

2. Infection, via transfer of micro-organisms
3. Particulate material being introduced, leading to inflammation
4. Bacterial endotoxins.

Buying instruments

All devices should be CE marked. The CE mark (officially CE marking) is a mandatory conformity mark on many products placed on the single market in the European Economic Area (EEA). The term initially used was 'EC mark' and it was officially replaced by 'CE marking' in the Directive 93/68/EEC in 1993. 'EC mark' is still in use, but is not the official term.

Specific custom-made instruments and new instruments undergoing evaluation may be the exception, but only with local authorisation and monitoring from a trust decontamination lead. Ophthalmic instruments are often extremely fragile and training in the care and maintenance of these particular instruments, for all those concerned with their decontamination, is crucial both to maintain their integrity and to avoid replacement costs.

55

Single-use instruments

NHS Estates (1999) recommended that, where possible, consideration should be given to using single-use devices.

Instruments marked by the manufacturer 'for single use only' should never be reused.

DECONTAMINATION STAGES

Cleaning

Cleaning is the most important stage in the decontamination process. Cleaning can be manual or mechanical depending on the instrument.

Disinfection

Disinfection is usually achieved by the use of liquid chemicals or by moist heat. Moist heat should be the method of choice except for devices unable to withstand high temperatures.

Inspection

Inspection of instruments should be performed by staff other than those responsible for cleaning them. Magnification should be used if possible for fine ophthalmic instruments. Damaged instruments should be removed for repair or disposal (after decontamination); inadequately cleaned items should be returned for further cleaning.

A final visual inspection should, however, always be made by the clinician before using any instrument.

Packaging

Some instruments will form part of sets of instruments and will be packed in trays; others will be packed singly in sealed pouches. All instruments must be traceable and the use of coloured tapes is not recommended because it may lead to inadequate decontamination. New instruments should be etched with a unique identifying code.

Sterilisation

The preferred method is the use of saturated steam under pressure, at the highest temperature compatible with the instruments being processed. Non-solid items and wrapped packs must be sterilised in autoclaves rather than in vacuum sterilisers. Benchtop sterilisers in theatres, clinics and primary care settings are being phased out because the cleaning and maintenance cycles, even with the best will, cannot be guaranteed.

Transportation

It is important that transport containers are waterproof, secure, labelled and protect both their contents and the handler.

Storage

Appropriate storage for these instruments is important. It should be above floor level and away from all sources of heat and water. In areas where instruments are not used frequently, storage should be 'in' rather than 'on' to avoid dust settlement on packaging.

NON-SURGICAL INSTRUMENTATION

No clinician can avoid leaving cell and other debris on tonometer heads, contact lenses and any other instrument that comes into contact with the eye or adnexae (Amin et al. 2003; Lim et al. 2003).

The guidelines of the Royal College of Ophthalmology (RCOphth; Hawksworth 2006: 6) state that:

> A solution containing 20,000 parts per million of available chlorine (sodium hypochlorite) is effective in reducing Transmissible Spongiform Encephalopathies, including vCJD. Soaking with 2% hypochlorite solution (e.g. Milton) between patients is therefore considered best decontamination practice.

Solutions should always be labelled to avoid inadvertent use.

TONOMETRY

Single-use options should be used whenever possible. It is obvious that single-use instrumentation should be used for patients who have, or are suspected of having, CJD; however, as this condition takes many years to develop, there is a good case for assuming that all patients potentially have transmissible infection – thus treating all patients in the same way.

Reusable tonometer prisms should not be allowed to dry after use; instead they should be washed and dried immediately, then wiped with alcohol and allowed to dry. After each session they should be washed and soaked in sodium hypochlorite (Hawksworth 2006).

DIAGNOSTIC CONTACT LENSES

Between patient examinations, diagnostic contact lenses should be washed clean while moist before immersion in 2% sodium hypochlorite solution (20 000 p.p.m.) for at least 5 min. Unless the solution is known to be eye safe, they should be rinsed in sterile saline and then dried.

To facilitate tracing, prisms and lenses should be moved around clinics and rooms as little as possible.

ENDOPHTHALMITIS

Postoperative endophthalmitis is a devastating complication of surgery. There are many processes in place to minimise the risk of endophthalmitis perioperatively; there are also a number of techniques used as prophylaxis against perioperative infection.

The most recent review of techniques concludes that only pre-operative povidone–iodine is 'moderately important to clinical outcome' (Ciulla et al. 2002). All other interventions that were revised (postoperative subconjunctival antibiotics, preoperative lash trimming, preoperative topical antibiotics, preoperative saline irrigation, irrigating solutions containing antibiotics and intraoperative heparin) receive a low clinical recommendation (possibly relevant to clinical outcome but not definitely linked) because of generally weak and conflicting evidence for their use.

Dealing with an outbreak of endophthalmitis

55

> The discovery or suspicion of an outbreak of endophthalmitis should prompt a rapid, systematic and open investigation to identify and eradicate the cause. Patient safety should be paramount and this may involve temporary cessation of intraocular surgery. (Elliott 2007: 5)

Comprehensive guidelines are available at: www.rcophth.ac.uk/docs/profstands/ophthalmicservices/EndophthalmitisJune2007.pdf

REFERENCES

Amin SZ, Smith L, Luthert PJ, Cheetham ME, Buckley RJ (2003). Minimizing the risk of prion transmission by contact tonometry. *Br J Ophthalmol* **87**:1360–2.

Ciulla TA, Starr MB, Masket S (2002). Bacterial endophthalmitis prophylaxis for cataract surgery: An evidence-based update. *Ophthalmology* **109**:13–24.

Department of Health (2007). *Report of the vCJD Clinical Governance Advisory Group*. London: DH. www.dh.gov.uk/en/Policyandguidance/Healthandsocialcaretopics/CJD/CJDgeneral-information/index.htm (accessed 28 June 2007).

Elliott A (2007). *Managing an Outbreak of Postoperative Endophthalmitis*. London: Royal College of Ophthalmologists.

Hawksworth N (2006). *Ophthalmic Instrument Decontamination*. London: Royal College of Ophthalmologists.

Jones NP (1998). *Uveitis: An illustrated manual*. Oxford: Butterworth-Heinemann.

Lankford MG, Zembower TR, Trick WE, Hacek DM, Noskin GA, Peterson LR (2003). Influence of role models and hospital design on hand hygiene of healthcare workers. *Emerging Infectious Diseases* **9**:217–23.

Lim R, Dhillon B, Kurian KM, Aspinall PA, Fernie K, Ironside JW (2003). Retention of corneal epithelial cells following Goldmann tonometry: implications for CJD. *Br J Ophthalmol* **87**:583–6.

NHS Estates (1999). *Variant Creutzfeldt–Jakob Disease (vCJD): Minimising the risk of transmission*. Health Service Circular HSC 1999/178. London: DH.

World Health Organization (2005). *Guidelines on Hand Hygiene in Health Care*. Geneva: WHO. Available at: www.cec.health.nsw.gov.au/pdf/WHOGuidelinesAdvancedDraft.pdf (accessed 23 October 2007).

55

FURTHER READING

Department of Health (2005). *Saving Lives: A delivery programme to reduce healthcare associated infection, including MRSA*. London: DH.

Department of Health (2006). *Standards for Better Health*. London: DH.

NHS Estates (2003). *A Guide to the Decontamination of Reusable Surgical Instruments*. London: DH.

Managing pain, nausea and vomiting

With ocular disease or trauma, pain is often the overriding feature that the patient complains of on presentation.

Differentiation of pain and its nature are often important in making a definitive diagnosis, for example, in acute angle-closure glaucoma that is frequently misdiagnosed in non-ophthalmic settings.

Following a review of the literature, Lee (1999) recommends the use of a pain assessment tool and the documentation of findings including how the pain was managed.

Pain assessment is an integral component of emergency triage and should always lead to the introduction of measures to alleviate that pain.

Instillation of topical anaesthetic should be routine at triage in all settings, for ocular surface pain. The triage nurse must therefore have a high level of knowledge about ophthalmic conditions and be able to recognise when the cause of pain is likely to be alleviated by topical anaesthetic and when other measures may be necessary.

Nausea and vomiting are a feature of some ophthalmic conditions such as angle-closure glaucoma as well as postoperatively (Waterman et al. 1999). In addition, some individuals from particular ethnic backgrounds have been found to experience nausea and vomiting after procedures such as fundus fluorescein angiography (FFA; McLaughlan et al. 1998).

In the case of FFA, the recommendation is that an antiemetic be given prophylactically where there has been previous nausea associated with the procedure and when the patient belongs to a susceptible group.

After oculoplastic procedures such as enucleation, studies have shown that there is a high incidence of pain as well as nausea and vomiting (Waterman et al. 1999). Waterman et al. recommend the prescribing of both oral analgesic agents and oral anti-inflammatory drugs and antiemetics.

As well as practically managing the patient medically, Waterman et al. (1999) recommend that consideration be given to the timing of discharge. When enucleation is performed, plan for an inpatient stay to include at least one full postoperative day in hospital. This allows the pain to be actively managed and controlled.

REFERENCES

Lee A (1999). Assessing ophthalmic pain using a verbal rating scale international. *J Ophthal Nursing* **2**(4):8–12.

McLaughlan R, Waterman H, Waterman C, Hillier V, Dodd C (1998). Ethnic variation in fluorescein angiography induced nausea and vomiting. *Eye* **12**(Pt 6):996–1000.

Waterman H, Leatherbarrow B, Slater R, Waterman C (1999). Postoperative pain, nausea and vomiting: qualitative perspectives from telephone interviews. *J Adv Nursing* **29**:690–6.

Visual acuity testing (in adults)   **57**

The word 'acuity' comes from the Latin *acuitas*, which means sharpness.

DEFINITION

Visual acuity (VA) is the acuteness or clarity of vision. This is dependent on the sharpness of the focus of the target object on the retina, the sensitivity of the nervous system and the ability of the brain to interpret the information (Cline et al. 1997). As such, any one or all of these systems being compromised can alter VA.

REASONS TO RECORD VA

All patients should undertake VA testing when practically possible depending upon initial presentation. This is a threefold necessity: first, to assess visual function on presentation, confirming subjective function on presentation; second and third, this initial record acts as a measure of regress or egress of conditions after treatment has been initiated.

HOW TO PERFORM VA TESTING (Snellen – Figure 57.1)

Visual acuity is typically measured monocularly rather than binocularly with the aid of an optotype chart for distant vision and an occluder to cover the eye not being tested. The examiner may also occlude an eye by instructing the patient to use his or her hand.

This latter method is typically avoided in clinical settings because it may inadvertently allow the patient to peek through his or her fingers, or press the eye and alter the measurement when that eye is evaluated.

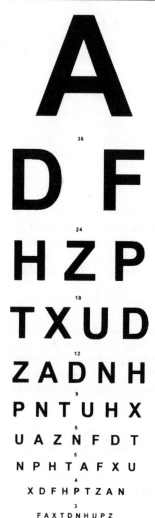

Figure 57.1 Snellen chart.

Place the chart at the correct distance (6 m or 3 m with a mirror) ensuring correct and appropriate luminosity.

If the patient uses distance glasses, the test is performed using them.

Place the occluder in front of the eye that is not being tested. The first tested eye is the one that is believed to see less or the one that the patient says is seeing less.

Start first at the top of the chart and ask the patient to read each letter in turn, working downwards to the smaller letters. The patient has to identify every letter on the line being presented and communicate it to the practitioner.

If the measurement is reduced (below 6/6) then the test using a pinhole should be done and the VA recorded using the pinhole. Both measures should be recorded, with and without using the pinhole.

Change the occluder to the other eye and proceed again from the top of the chart.

After both eyes have been evaluated in distant VA, proceed to evaluate near VA using a 'near book'.

Difficulties may arise with patients having limited understanding of the letter symbols (optotypes) on the chart used if they do not have knowledge of English. However, there are alternative methods for VA testing, less reliant on optotypes: for example, Illiterate (or Tumbling) E Test and Landholt C tests. A tactful approach to patients with reading problems should be used and the use of a matching chart (where the patient is provided with a page of large letters and asked to match them to the letter on the distant testing chart) is preferable to the use of child-specific charts for adults. Translators should not be used for VA testing because they may bias the outcome by false reporting (Shaw 2006).

Snellen and similar charts have disadvantages in that there are a different number of letters at each level. Spacing of letters and progression of letter size is uneven so the visual task is not the same at each level of acuity. LogMAR charts have been developed to address theses issues. MAR stands for 'minimum angle of resolution', which is the minutes of degrees broken into smaller sections. This is converted into a logarithm known as logMAR.

LOGMAR CHARTS (Figure 57.2)

Charts are designed with the same number of letters on each row, similar spacing between letters and consistent spacing between rows. Testing takes place at 4 m, a distance much more manageable than 6 m in most clinic settings. The test takes place in the same way as for Snellen testing. The patient should be encouraged to read from left to right and to continue down the chart until he or she fails to see any letters on a line. Every letter **missed** or **read incorrectly** is taken into account when noting visual acuity – each letter equals 0.1 log unit each line. The chart is marked with logMAR notation on one side and Snellen on the other; the value of 0.0 logMAR is equivalent to 4/4 Snellen (or 6/6). Each line on the chart is 0.1 logMAR and therefore each letter is 0.02. The total number of letters missed or incorrect is noted and a score of 0.02 for each added to the logMAR value for the last line on which any letter was read correctly. This becomes the final score.

RECORDING SNELLEN VA

The numerator is the distance that the patient is from the chart. The denominator is the line to which the patient reads. Incom-

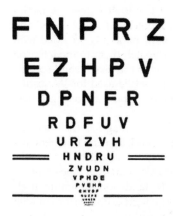

Figure 57.2 LogMAR.

plete lines can be added to the last complete line, for example, 6/12 + 3, indicating that the patient read the 12 lines at 6 m and gained 3 random letters on line 9.

If VA is so poor that the patient cannot recognise the optotype, the next measurement is counting fingers (CF), followed by hand movements (HM), then perception of light (PL) and finally no perception of light (NPL).

6/6 OR 20/20?

6/6 is the UK equivalent of 20/20.

The numerator of 6 indicates that the person is 6 m from the chart, which equates to 20 feet in the USA.

VA CONVERSION SCALES

Snellen notation		MAR	LogMAR	Decimal
UK	USA			
6/60	20/200	10	1.0	0.10
6/48	20/160	8.0	0.9	0.13
6/38	20/125	6.3	0.8	0.16
6/30	20/100	5.0	0.7	0.20
6/24	20/80	4.0	0.6	0.25
6/19	20/60	3.2	0.5	0.32
6/15	20/50	2.5	0.4	0.40
6/12	20/40	2.0	0.3	0.50
6/9.5	20/30	1.6	0.2	0.63
6/7.5	20/25	1.25	0.1	0.80
6/6	20/20	1.00	0.0	1.00
6/4.8	20/16	0.80	−0.1	1.25
6/3.8	20/12.5	0.63	−0.2	1.58
6/3.0	20/10	0.50	−0.3	2.00

From Bailey and Lovie (1976).

REFERENCES

Bailey IL, Lovie JE (1976). New design principles for visual acuity letter charts. *Am J Optom Physiol Opt* **53**:740–5.

Cline D, Hofstetter HW, Griffin JR (1997). *Dictionary of Visual Science*, 4th edn. Boston, MA: Butterworth-Heinemann.

Shaw M (2006). Examination of the eye. In: Marsden J (ed.), *Ophthalmic Care*. Chichester: Wiley, 66–84.

Section 11

Legal aspects of care and policy

Low vision registration

The Government launched a new system for registering people as blind or partially sighted in England in November 2003. This was revised in August 2005. Registers are held by Social Services Departments of local councils or by voluntary organisations on their behalf. Registration remains optional but services can be put in place for those not eligible for registration or those who do not wish to be registered

New standard referral documents should be available from optometrists and the hospital eye service to request help for people with visual impairment from Social Services. These documents may be used before registration, or even if the person decides not to register.

The Low Vision Leaflet (LVL)

This is an information guide for patients that gives contact details for information, advice and help; it has a tear-off form that the person can fill in and send to local Social Services to ask for a low vision assessment. This replaces the Letter of Visual Impairment, which was introduced at the start of the changes to the process in 2003.

Referral of Vision Impairment (RVI)

In the eye unit, staff can fill in an RVI form, which will inform Social Services about the patient's situation and need for support, and request an assessment. This can be done for patients who are not eligible for registration, but are in need of help and support. The urgency of assessment can be stated, which should help Social Services to prioritise.

Certificate of Vision Impairment (CVI)

The BD8 has been replaced by the CVI, which, as for the BD8, must be filled in by a consultant ophthalmologist to notify Social Services that someone is eligible for registration and trigger an assessment of needs.

The CVI is available only in an electronic, downloadable form. Hospital eye services are able to download it from the NHSweb at: www.doh.nhs01.nhs.uk/nhsweb/nhskbweb.nsf/0/1E12A4E3CFE6B27380256F4200409D07?OpenDocument

A version can be viewed by those who do not have access to NHSweb at: www.dh.gov.uk/PolicyAndGuidance/HealthAnd SocialCareTopics/Optical/fs/en

When registration is complete, a registration card is offered to the patient to confirm registration.

CHANGES TO TERMINOLOGY

For registration purposes, the term 'blind' now becomes 'severely sight impaired (blind)' and 'partially sighted' becomes 'sight impaired (partially sighted)'.

Social Services

There are current performance indicators that apply to older clients and the Department of Health (DH 2005) suggests that the following would be best practice:

- The time from first contact to the beginning of assessment should be ≤48 h.
- After the completion of assessment, all services in the care package should have been supplied within 28 days. If this 'package' includes a rehabilitation programme, this should be well under way (at least two sessions) with no planned interruption before its completion.

In general, Social Services aim for initial contact to be within 10 working days to establish the urgency of the need and to give information about statutory and voluntary services.

Entitlement to benefits

The University of Central England and the Royal National Institute for the Blind (RNIB) (2005) have produced a guide to benefits, summarised here.

Anyone with a visual disability is entitled to the following, whether registered or not:

- Support from Social Services
- Low vision aids
- Railcard and other rail travel concessions
- Disability Living Allowance (DLA)
- Attendance Allowance (AA)
- Incapacity Benefit
- Additional Income Support or Pension Credit
- Housing Benefit or Council Tax Benefit
- Protection under the Disability Discrimination Act (DDA) legislation
- Protection under Special Educational Needs and Disability Act (SENDA) 2001 legislation
- Working Tax Credit.

Only people registered as Severely Sight Impaired or Sight Impaired are entitled to:

- Free NHS eye tests
- Free NHS prescriptions
- Free directory enquiries
- Disabled Person's Parking (Blue) Badge
- Disabled Person's Tax Credit
- Access to Work scheme
- Radio, cassette or CD player.

Only people registered Severely Sight Impaired are entitled to:

- Additional Personal Income Tax Allowance
- Reduction in television licence fee.

REFERENCES

Department of Health (2005). *The Identification, Referral and Registration of Sight Loss: Action for Social Services departments and optometrists, and explanatory notes.* London: DH.

University of Central England, RNIB (2005). *Entitlement to Benefit.* Available at: www.sightlossmatters.com

USEFUL CONTACTS
www.rnib.org.uk
RNIB Welfare Rights team: 0845 766
Government Benefits Enquiry Line: 0800 882200

Recommendations for low vision services (NHS Eyecare Services Programme, RNIB 2007)

59

A low vision service is a rehabilitative process that provides a range of services for people with low vision to enable them to make best use of their eyesight and visual function to achieve maximum potential.

DESIGN PRINCIPLES

1. Low vision services should reflect a multidisciplinary, multi-agency approach that coordinates with other health-care, social care and voluntary providers in the area, including services provided at the client's residence, school or other appropriate location.
2. The services delivered should be based upon needs identified by clients and/or carers and be flexible enough to meet the disparate needs of its client group, including those with additional disabilities. There should be evidence of user participation in agreements on the development and implementation of pathways and protocols.
3. Registration as sight impaired or severely sight impaired should not be a prerequisite to accessing services.
4. Locally designed guidelines, pathways and protocols should be underpinned, whenever possible, by evidence-based knowledge and accepted guidance. This should conform with and contribute to governance arrangements for health care and social care.
5. Timescales should be agreed and monitored, by all parties.

59

- Each part of the process should be subject to an appropriate booking procedure.
- The client should be advised of current waiting times along with highlighted 'not later than' times/dates.
- Contact should ideally be made within 10 working days.

  Note that local commissioners and service providers will need to identify acceptable timescales for each stage of the protocol/care pathway. Timescales recommended Standard 8.5 (ADSS 2002) are for clients to be seen within 10 working days of referral or receiving their CVI, RVI or LVL (see previous chapter).

- A client's low vision needs should be reviewed as appropriate. Regular eye examinations should be recommended.

The following is an example of what clients may require. Initial action upon referral to low vision services:

- Provision of information about and description of the service, outline of the processes involved and what is likely to happen.
- Access to help, advice and support line, ensuring that appropriate formats and languages used (national or local service).
- Details of current waiting times.
- Booking of appointments at each stage of the process. Clients should be informed of the duration of each stage of the process.
- Access to counselling (this may be urgent and in advance of the low vision assessment).
- Provision of a single contact point for information on all aspects of the service, irrespective of where a client may be on the care pathway.

REFERRAL, ASSESSMENT AND SERVICE

6. Referral to low vision services should be open to any healthcare or social care professional based upon locally developed guidance. This should also include self-referral and subsequent requests for review.

The guidance should be devised with input from local professionals including ophthalmologists, optometrists, dispensing opticians, ophthalmic nurses, orthoptists, occupational therapists, general practitioners, rehabilitation workers, Social Services, voluntary services, potential users and others.

7. Clients should be able to access the service irrespective of the degree of sight loss or reduction in vision, as early as possible, to minimise negative impact on quality of life. The definition of a person with low vision is one who has an impairment of visual function for whom full remediation is not possible by conventional spectacles, contact lenses, or medical or surgical intervention, and which causes restriction in that person's everyday life. The perception of what constitutes a restriction in a person's everyday life will vary from individual to individual. Access to the service should therefore not be based on clinical or social criteria.

8. It is essential that there is a diagnosis of the associated eye and/or systemic condition(s). Practitioners should ensure that all appropriate medical interventions are being or have been employed, and patients must be given appropriate and understandable information about the importance of an eye examination, as well as their condition. Diagnosis can occur either before or simultaneous with accessing the low vision service.

   Clients may refuse to be referred to another professional at any stage of the process, even if informed that it is in their best interests. Records should be documented accordingly and the client informed that he or she could still proceed with referral at a later date.

9. There should be a tailored low vision assessment for each client following referral:
   - At the point of initial contact with low vision services an appropriate and comprehensive range of services available should be discussed or highlighted, using appropriate methods. Clients should discuss whether they wish to be considered for all of them or be facilitated to choose to access those that they feel are appropriate. If a service is

declined at any stage, this should not preclude clients from being offered and/or accepting it at a later stage.

- Once a client has been referred, a full assessment of their needs should be undertaken by means of an appropriate comprehensive low vision service. A care and delivery plan can then be agreed with the client. After initial assessment it will be necessary to review the range of services to consider appropriateness and whether other services might be indicated.

10. A low vision assessment should always offer:
    - An eye health examination, evidence of recent examination or referral for examination.
    - A functional visual assessment.

11. The following should be offered, as appropriate to the user, after assessment:
    - Prescription/provision of appropriate optical/non-optical aids.
    - Advice on lighting, contrast and size, filters, tactile aids, electronic aids and other non-optical aids.
    - Training and/or therapy to enable optical and non-optical aids and other techniques to be used effectively.
    - Links to broader rehabilitation services and referral to structured therapy programmes, counselling, education and employment services.
    - A review of benefits, welfare rights, concessions, and both local and national support groups.

INFORMATION

12. Information should be provided in a format that is appropriate to the need of each client. The information should enable clients to make informed decisions about their care.

13. Information should be communicated to other professionals involved in client care and the referral source with appropriate prior consent from the client. Information should be in an accessible format for all individuals.

14. All professionals interacting with a client within a low vision service should use a health-care record, which can be shared with appropriate prior consent from the client.

SERVICE IMPROVEMENT, MONITORING AND EVALUATION OF
THE SERVICE

15. Local commissioners will wish to ensure that service improvement, modernisation techniques and learning from related areas are considered, implemented and evaluated. It is also important to have in place appropriate measures and recording systems to identify the current position, have on-going information about number of people referred and treated, client demographics and interprofessional communications, as well as provision of data to allow evaluation of the service. Service users should be involved.

16. Local commissioners should ideally be working towards producing an evidence-based, concise, annual report on the service, available in the public domain.

TRAINING

17. All people who wish to participate in the delivery of the service should be suitably trained or undergo a training programme agreed locally as part of the protocol. Training should lead to accreditation to participate in the scheme. The training programme should be designed to ensure quality and a seamless service between health care and social care. It should also include knowledge of working with people who have learning, communication and multiple disabilities.

    A mechanism for ongoing accreditation should be built into the training programme.

    Training should be of a multidisciplinary nature, ensuring that all those involved understand the different and related roles.

18. It is good practice for commissioners to ensure that all personnel involved in the service with sole access to clients should have an appropriate check carried out by the Criminal Records Bureau.

19. The client should expect that information relating to their health or welfare should be respected and remain confidential between personnel within the service, unless disclosure is specifically permitted by the client or is required by law.

LIST OF BENEFITS AND SERVICES AT THE TIME OF PUBLICATION, JANUARY 2007

Benefit or assistance	Severely sight impaired	Sight impaired
Pension Credit, Housing Benefit, Council Tax Benefit	Based on income	Based on income
Additional Income Support	Yes	Yes
Additional Pension Credit	Yes	Yes
Blind Person's Personal Income Tax Allowance	Yes	N/A
Disability Living Allowance (≤64)	Yes	Yes
Attendance Allowance (≥65)	Yes	Yes
Additional Housing Benefit or Council Tax Benefit	Yes	Possible
Exemption from non-dependants' deduction from Income Support	Yes	Possible
Council tax reduction	Yes	Yes
Incapacity Benefit	Yes	Yes
Working Tax Credit	Yes	Yes
Financial help towards residential/ nursing home fees	Possible	Possible
Community care services/local council assistance	Yes	Yes
NHS sight test	Yes	Yes
NHS prescription	Possible	Possible
TV licence reduction	Yes	N/A
Car parking Blue Badge scheme	Yes	Possible
Access to work equipment	Yes	Yes
Articles for the Blind Postage	Yes	Yes
Railcard	Yes	Yes
Local travel concessions	Possible	Possible
Free directory enquiries	Yes	Yes

Benefit or assistance	Severely sight impaired	Sight impaired
British Wireless for the Blind	Yes	**N/A**
Telephone installation charge and line rental	Yes	**N/A**
Low vision assessment	Possible	Possible
Low vision aids	Possible	Possible
RNIB Talking Books	Yes	Yes
Big print newspaper	Yes	Yes
Calibre	Yes	Yes
Postal lending library	Yes	Yes
Talking Newspapers Association UK	Yes	Yes
Local Talking Newspapers	Yes	Yes
Talk and support	Yes	Yes

Note that 'possible' indicates that may be available according to individual circumstance and/or local arrangements. N/A, not available.

The material in this chapter is reproduced with permission of the Department of Health.

REFERENCES

Assistant Directors of Social Services (2002). *Progress in Sight – National standards of social care for visually impaired adults.* London: ADSS.

NHS Eyecare Services Programme/Royal National Institute for the Blind (2007). *Recommended Standards for Low Vision Services.* London: DH.

59

Consent provides the only lawful justification for treatment. There is no legal requirement that consent should be written, or be in a particular form – oral consent is valid (or it may be implied from circumstances, where, for example, a patient holds out an arm to have venepuncture). However, a written consent form provides evidence of consent and is recommended for anything other than very minor procedures.

If valid consent is not given, any treatment that involves touching – for example, physical examination, surgery, taking blood specimens – would amount to battery.

Consent is not a one-off procedure but is continuous throughout any patient episode and the clinician must ensure that the patient knows all that is happening at every stage of treatment and care, and is aware that consent may be withdrawn at any time.

In fact consent can be withdrawn, even after signing a consent form, and to proceed with treatment where consent has effectively been withdrawn also constitutes battery.

For consent to be valid it must be:

- given by someone who is competent (has legal capacity)
- sufficiently informed
- freely given.

REQUIREMENTS FOR INFORMED CONSENT

The General Medical Council (GMC) provides a comprehensive set of guidelines for doctors obtaining consent. They state:

> You must be satisfied that you have consent or other valid authority before you undertake any examination or

investigation, provide treatment or involve patients in teaching or research. Usually this will involve providing information to patients in a way they can understand, before asking for their consent. (GMC 2006: 20)

This guidance is relevant to all clinicians who are obtaining consent for any procedure. They suggest that information that the patient ought to know before deciding to consent to investigation or treatment might include:

- the diagnosis and prognosis and likely prognosis if the condition is not treated
- any uncertainties about the diagnosis and options for further investigation
- management options
- the purpose of proposed treatment or investigation with details of the procedure and any other therapies included such as pain relief
- preparation and likely experiences of the procedure
- benefits, probabilities of success, serious or frequently occurring risks, and effects on life and lifestyle of all procedures
- who will be undertaking the procedure and how doctors in training will be supervised
- a reminder that the patient can change his or her mind at any point and also, that the patient has a right to seek a second opinion.

The GMC also stresses that this should all be done in a way that the patient understands, using appropriate language and materials.

Clinicians cannot carry out procedures for which the patient has not consented, except in an emergency, and any likely emergency procedures should be explored beforehand so that the patient can specifically consent, or withhold consent to them.

Information that is relevant to decision-making should never be withheld unless:

. . . you judge that disclosure of some relevant information would cause the patient serious harm. In this context serious harm does not mean the patient would become upset, or decide to refuse treatment. (GMC 1998)

Where a relative wishes the clinician to withhold information, the clinician should seek the views of the patient and only withhold relevant information as stated above.

It is difficult sometimes to inform patients fully of the options because it appears that they do not want to know and would rather the clinician did what he or she felt best. This is not an option. Patients cannot nominate others to make decisions for them and basic information must be provided, even if the more complex details are not discussed.

If, in any circumstances, information is withheld from the patient, it should be fully documented with the justification for the decision made in the patient's notes.

The GMC (2006) again give very good guidance that is reproduced here.

The clinician should:

- use up-to-date written material, visual and other aids to explain complex aspects of the investigation, diagnosis or treatment where appropriate and/or practicable
- make arrangements, wherever possible, to meet particular language and communication needs, for example, through translations, independent interpreters, signers or the patient's representative
- where appropriate, discuss with patients the possibility of bringing a relative or friend, or making a tape recording of the consultation
- explain the probabilities of success, or the risk of failure of, or harm associated with, options for treatment, using accurate data
- ensure that information that patients may find distressing is given to them in a considerate way
- provide patients with information about counselling services and patient support groups, where appropriate
- allow patients sufficient time to reflect, before and after making a decision, especially where the information is complex or the

severity of the risks is great; where patients have difficulty understanding information, or there is a lot of information to absorb, it may be appropriate to provide it in manageable amounts, with appropriate written or other back-up material, over a period of time, or to repeat it

- involve nursing or other members of the health-care team in discussions with the patient, where appropriate; they may have valuable knowledge of the patient's background or particular concerns, for example, in identifying what risks the patient should be told about
- ensure, where treatment is not to start until some time after consent has been obtained, that the patient is given a clear route for reviewing the decision with the person providing the treatment.

WHO CAN TAKE CONSENT?

People who take consent should be those who are carrying out the procedure, or someone delegated by them whom they know. The person should:

- be suitably trained and qualified
- have sufficient knowledge of the investigation or treatment and understand all the risks involved
- act in accordance with best practice (GMC 2006).

CAPACITY TO CONSENT

Two Acts of Parliament have a bearing on capacity to consent: the Mental Capacity Act 2005 is in place in England and Wales, and the Adults with Incapacity (Scotland) Act 2000 in Scotland. There is currently no equivalent law on mental capacity in Northern Ireland but the Bamford Review of Mental Health and Learning Disability is looking at how current law affects people with mental health needs or a learning disability in Northern Ireland.

The Mental Capacity Act 2005

For the purposes of this Act, a person lacks capacity in relation to a matter if at the material time he is unable to make a decision for himself in relation to the matter because of an impairment of, or a disturbance in the functioning of, the mind or brain.

It does not matter whether the impairment or disturbance is permanent or temporary and the question of whether or not the person lacks capacity must be decided on the balance of probabilities. The Act applies only to those aged over 16.

The person is unable to make a decision if he or she is unable to:

- understand the information relevant to the decision
- retain that information; if he or she can retain the information for a period long enough to make a decision, the decision is valid
- use the information as part of the process of making the decision
- communicate the decision.

The information must be given in a way that is appropriate for the person and may include simple language, visual aids, sign language, etc.

If asked to act in the best interests of the person, all factors should be taken into account and the person taking consent should try to find out the patient's past and present wishes, feelings and beliefs, and values that might impact on the decision. Account should also be taken of the views of anyone named by the person as someone to be consulted, anyone caring for the person, anyone with Enduring Power of Attorney and anyone appointed by the court to look after the interests of the person. However, the clinician should then act in the best interests of the patient. All aspects of this process should be documented.

Adults with Incapacity (Scotland) Act 2000
This Act is similar in that it states that:

Any intervention in the affairs of an incapacitated adult must:

60

- benefit the adult;

- take account of the adult's wishes, so far as these can be ascertained;

- take account of the views of relevant others, as far as it is reasonable and practical to do so; and

- restrict the adult's freedom as little as possible while still achieving the desired benefit.

It introduces a certificate of incapacity that must be issued in order to provide care or treatment where there is no proxy decision-maker for the person (or in the case of an emergency). Once this has been issued, doctors have a general authority to treat the person.

Proxy consent may be given on behalf of an incapacitated adult by a welfare attorney or appointed welfare guardian with powers relating to the treatment in question. The proxy may also refuse treatment as long as he or she is doing so in the best interests of the person.

CHILDREN AND CONSENT

In law, children are those who are under 18 years of age. For the purposes of giving consent to treatment, children are treated differently in law according to their age.

The Family Reform Act 1969 provides that the consent to treatment of a 16 or 17 year old is to be treated like the consent of an adult.

For those children aged under 16 there is precedent in case law governing consent to treatment (*Gillick v West Norfolk and Wisbech AHA* 1986).

This states that, if a minor has sufficient intelligence and understanding to enable him or her to understand the treatment and implications of treatment, then he or she is 'Gillick competent' and can consent to treatment.

For babies, young children and older children who are not competent in law, someone else must consent on their behalf.

This can be a proxy or, occasionally, the court. A proxy is generally a parent or another person with parental responsibility. In making a decision about medical treatment the proxy must act in the child's best interests. Usually consent should be obtained only from one parent, although, if the two parents disagree, the courts are often involved. If there is a difference of opinion between the parent and the clinician, again the court should be involved. In an emergency situation, where a parent cannot be contacted, the child can be treated without consent, but only where treatment is immediately necessary.

A child who is competent can consent to treatment. However, a refusal of treatment may be overridden by a parent or the court, when such a refusal would be likely to result in the death or permanent disability of the child. The wishes of the child may be overridden to preserve his or her long-term interests.

CONSENT FORMS

The four forms are designed to meet the needs of different groups of patients:

1. Consent form 1 for patients able to consent for themselves.
2. Consent form 2 for those with parental responsibility, consenting on behalf of a child/young person.
3. Consent form 3 both for patients able to consent for themselves and for those with parental responsibility consenting on behalf of a child/young person, where the procedure does not involve any impairment of consciousness. As the patient is expected to remain alert during the procedure, some of the information covered in forms 1 and 2 is unnecessary. The use of this form is optional.
4. Consent form 4 for adults who lack capacity to consent to a particular treatment. This form requires health professionals to document both how they have come to the conclusion that the patient lacks capacity and why the proposed treatment is in the patient's best interests. It also allows the involvement of those close to the patient in making this health-care decision to be documented.

60

CONSEQUENCES OF LACK OF CONSENT

Battery

Battery is any non-consensual touching – it does not have to harm the patient. A clinician can commit battery even though he or she feels that he or she is acting in the patient's best interests. To avoid liability in battery the patient needs to be aware of what is about to happen and give consent for it.

Negligence

If patients do not feel that they have been sufficiently informed about the treatment or the risks inherent in it, they can then claim for negligence. In deciding whether lack of disclosure is negligent, it is necessary to determine what the responsible body of clinicians in that particular field would have disclosed (the Bolam test – *Bolam v Friern Hospital Management Committee* 1957). Cases have been deemed negligent where disclosure has not taken place when:

- the incidence of the risk is sufficiently high
- the consequences of the risk happening would be serious for the patient
- the patient specifically asks about a risk (www.ethics-network. org.uk).

REFUSAL OF TREATMENT

Adults

A competent adult may refuse treatment even if the consequences of lack of treatment would be severe (even if the patient's life depended on the treatment). This applies to all competent adults.

> The patient is entitled to reject [the] advice for reasons which are rational, or irrational, or for no reason. (Per Lord Templeman in *Sidaway v Board of Governors of Bethlem Royal Hospital* 1985)

BOX 60.1 TWELVE KEY POINTS ON CONSENT: THE LAW IN
ENGLAND (WWW.DOH.GOV.UK/CONSENT)

When do health professionals need consent from patients?
 1. Before you examine, treat or care for competent adult
    patients you must obtain their consent.
 2. Adults are always assumed to be competent unless
    demonstrated otherwise. If you have doubts about their
    competence, the question to ask is: 'Can this patient
    understand and weigh up the information needed to
    make this decision?' Unexpected decisions do not prove
    that the patient is incompetent, but may indicate a need
    for further information or explanation.
 3. Patients may be competent to make some health-care
    decisions, even if they are not competent to make others.
 4. Giving and obtaining consent is usually a process, not a
    one-off event. Patients can change their minds and
    withdraw consent at any time. If there is any doubt, you
    should always check that the patient still consents to
    your caring for or treating them.

Can children give consent for themselves?
 5. Before examining, treating or caring for a child, you
    must also seek consent. Young people aged 16 and 17
    are presumed to have the competence to give consent
    for themselves. Younger children who understand fully
    what is involved in the proposed procedure can also
    give consent (although their parents will ideally be
    involved). In other cases, someone with parental
    responsibility must give consent on the child's behalf,

60

unless they cannot be reached in an emergency. If a competent child consents to treatment, a parent cannot override that consent. Legally, a parent can consent if a competent child refuses, but it is likely that taking such a serious step will be rare.

Who is the right person to seek consent?

6. It is always best for the person actually treating the patient to seek the patient's consent. However, you may seek consent on behalf of colleagues if you are capable of performing the procedure in question, or if you have been specially trained to seek consent for that procedure.

What information should be provided?

7. Patients need sufficient information before they can decide whether to give their consent: for example, information about the benefits and risks of the proposed treatment, and alternative treatments. If the patient is not offered as much information as is reasonably needed to make the decision, and in a form that he or she can understand, the consent may not be valid.

8. Consent must be given voluntarily: not under any form of duress or undue influence from health professionals, family or friends.

Does it matter how the patient gives consent?

9. No: consent can be written, oral or non-verbal. A signature on a consent form does not itself prove that the consent is valid – the point of the form is to record the patient's decision, and also increasingly the discussions that have taken place. Your trust or organisation may have a policy setting out when you need to obtain written consent.

Refusal of treatment

10. Competent adult patients are entitled to refuse treatment, even when it would clearly benefit their health. The only exception to this rule is where the treatment is for a mental disorder and the patient is

detained under the Mental Health Act 1983. A competent pregnant woman may refuse any treatment, even if this would be detrimental to the fetus.

Adults who are not competent to give consent

11. No-one can give consent on behalf of an incompetent adult. However, you may still treat such a patient if the treatment would be in their best interests. 'Best interests' go wider than best medical interests, to include factors such as the wishes and beliefs of the patient when competent, and the patient's current wishes, general well-being, and spiritual and religious welfare. People close to the patient may be able to give you information on some of these factors. Where the patient has never been competent, relatives, carers and friends may be best placed to advise on the patient's needs and preferences.

12. If an incompetent patient has clearly indicated in the past, while competent, that he or she would refuse treatment in certain circumstances (an 'advance refusal'), and those circumstances arise, you must abide by that refusal.

From Department of Health (2001).

REFERENCES

Department of Health (2001). *Twelve Key Points on Consent: The law in England.* London: DH. Available at: www.doh.gov.uk/consent

General Medical Council (1998). *Seeking Patients' Consent: The ethical considerations.* London: GMC. Available at: www.ethics-network.org.uk/Ethics/econsent.htm#guidelines

General Medical Council (2006). *Good Medical Practice.* London: GMC.

Vision and driving

The single most important sense for driving is vision. It is estimated that the driver receives up to 90% of the information needed to carry out this task safely through the visual system. Standards exist so that at some point along the continuum between very poor, or no, vision and perfect vision a person is deemed fit to drive.

In the UK, the single test of visual ability to drive is undertaken at the time of the driving test. The law states that the driver must be able to read (with correction if required) a registration plate, attached to a vehicle, with letters 79 mm high and 57 mm wide at a distance of 20.5 m (if the vehicle was registered before September 2001 or letters 50 mm wide at 20 m if registered during or after September 2001, equating to around 6/10 acuity) (Driver and Vehicle Licensing Authority or DVLA – www.dvla.gov.uk). This test is not open to interpretation and drivers who fail it are committing an offence under the Road Traffic Act 1988.

A defined field of vision is required for driving but is not tested for routinely, assuming that everyone taking a driving test has a normal field of vision.

This is the only test that a driver in the UK is likely to take to assess their vision for driving unless they come to the attention of the DVLA for some reason, until their driving licence needs renewing at age 70. Even then, drivers often tell their GPs that they are fit and GPs sign the necessary forms. Visual acuity does not need to be assessed.

Drivers in the UK are obliged to report any change in their circumstances, such as eye disease or injury, to the DVLA so that a decision can be made about fitness to drive.

Although the standard for the UK appears clear, Currie et al. (2000) found that 26% of patients with 6/9 vision failed the number plate test, and 34% with 6/12 vision passed it. They also found that optometric, ophthalmology and GP advice on whether or not the person could drive was inconsistent.

The regulations are divided into two groups, corresponding to licence type.

A group 1 licence includes cars, motor cycles and light goods vehicles, whereas a group 2 licence includes large (previously heavy) goods vehicles (LGVs), passenger-carrying vehicles (PCVs), medium goods vehicles and minibuses.

Table 61.1 Visual standards for driving

	Group 1 entitlement	**Group 2 entitlement**
Visual acuity	Able to meet the number plate test	New applicants are barred if the acuity using corrective lenses is worse than 6/9 in the better eye or 6/12 in the other eye. Uncorrected acuity must be at least 3/60 (some grandfather rights apply)
Monocular vision	Complete loss of vision in one eye. The person must inform the DVLA but will be able to drive when advised that he or she has adapted to the disability, acuity in the remaining eye fulfils the requirement and there is a normal monocular field in the remaining eye	Complete loss of an eye or vision of less than 3/60 uncorrected in one eye. Applicants are barred from holding a group 2 licence

61

Table 61.1 Continued

	Group 1 entitlement	**Group 2 entitlement**
Visual field defects glaucoma, retinopathy, retinitis pigmentosa, hemianopia, etc.	Driving must cease unless the person is confirmed as able to have a field of at least 120° on the horizon measured using a target equivalent to the white Goldmann 1114e setting. There should be no significant defect in the binocular field that encroaches within 20° of fixation above or below the horizontal meridian	A normal binocular field of vision is required Some grandfather rights apply for those who had a licence before 1/1/91
Diplopia	Cease driving on diagnosis – resumption on confirmation to the DVLA that diplopia is controlled by glasses or a patch that the driver undertakes to wear while driving. In exceptional cases, a stable diplopia may be compatible with driving, with consultant support	Permanent refusal or revocation of licence. Patching is not acceptable
Night blindness	Cases considered on an individual basis	Cases considered on an individual basis
Colour blindness	Need not notify the DVLA	Need not notify the DVLA
Blepharospasm	Consultant opinion is required. Control with botulinum toxin may be acceptable	Consultant opinion is required. Control with botulinum toxin may be acceptable

Modified from Marsden (2006).

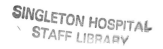

Patients with neurological problems such as stroke should have field testing because homonymous or bitemporal field defects that come close to fixation are a bar to driving. Certain static defects that have been present for a long time may be considered as exceptional cases. For some holders of group 2 licences, grandfather rights apply and type 2 licences obtained before the more stringent regulations came into force were not revoked.

PEOPLE WHO SHOULD NOT BE DRIVING

It is likely that clinicians will encounter people who should not be driving. Temporary visual impairment is much easier to deal with than permanent impairment because the loss of independence resulting from the loss of a driving licence may be a very difficult concept for the patient to come to terms with.

Padding

People wearing an eyepad should not drive. They have been rendered monocular and the regulations state that people who are monocular should not drive until they have adapted to the disability. Their licence to drive is compromised by this change and their insurance may be invalid because the insurance company has not been apprised of the change in visual status. They are therefore liable to prosecution as a result of an invalid licence and insurance. There are few occasions where patients have to be padded, and it is much easier to facilitate their journey home without a pad than run the risk of the danger to themselves and others while driving.

Dilatation

The only standard for driving in the UK is the number plate test, which may be carried out by police at the roadside. It must, however, be attached to a motor vehicle. A dilated pupil does not affect the patient's distance visual acuity and therefore they are likely to be able to fulfil the requirements for driving. A recent study (Potamitis et al. 2000) suggested that pupillary dilatation may lead to a decrease in vision and daylight driving performance in young people but considered a sample of only 12 people. At present, therefore, there is no regulation that stops people with dilated pupils from driving, although they should be warned about glare and lack of accommodation and that, if they do not feel able to drive, they should not. Insurance companies may take a different view of driving while dilated and the patient must be informed of this when making the decision whether or not to drive with dilated pupils.

Reduced acuity caused by lack of correction

Patients should be informed that, without correction, they do not have visual acuity of a legal standard for driving. The legal aspects of driving should be highlighted along with the consequences for insurance and the safety of other road users.

Visual acuity and field loss

It is the driver's responsibility to inform the DVLA of any changes in visual function. The clinician has a problem if the patient/driver refuses. Patient confidentiality undoubtedly applies and the clinician should not, without a great deal of consideration and multidisciplinary discussion, inform the DVLA unilaterally. That discussion should be recorded in the patient's notes along with any decisions made. The patient should be informed and given the opportunity to inform the DVLA before clinician involvement.

REFERENCES

Currie Z, Bhan A, Pepper I (2000). Reliability of Snellen charts for testing visual acuity for driving: prospective study and postal questionnaire. *BMJ* **321**:990–2.

Marsden J (2006). *Ophthalmic Care.* Chichester: Wiley.

Potamitis T, Slade SV, Fitt AW et al. (2000). The effect of pupil dilation with tropicamide on vision and driving simulator performance. *Eye* **14**:302–6.

Standards for information for people with a visual disability

Independent access to information is a fundamental need in health care. Blind or partially sighted people who cannot read instructions or information have to choose between asking someone else to read it to them and doing without the information. This compromises confidentiality, personal safety and dignity.

Not only is it unfair and potentially dangerous to discriminate against those with visual disability, but it is also unlawful not to meet their information needs. The Disability Discrimination Act 1995 states that:

19. (1) It is unlawful for a provider of services to discriminate against a disabled person:

(a) in refusing to provide, or deliberately not providing, to the disabled person any service which he provides, or is prepared to provide, to members of the public;

(b) in failing to comply with any duty imposed on him by section 21 in circumstances in which the effect of that failure is to make it impossible or unreasonably difficult for the disabled person to make use of any such service;

(c) in the standard of service which he provides to the disabled person or the manner in which he provides it to him; or

(d) in the terms on which he provides a service to the disabled person.

On 25 April 2007, the Royal National Institute for the Blind (RNIB) launched a series of leaflets called 'Information is Power'. The leaflet on health suggests five priorities for action:

1. Record the format that service users require for information, such as appointments, treatment and test results, and ensure that future information distribution is provided in this format.
2. Ensure that there is a full understanding of the information needs of blind and partially sighted patients outlined within the Disability Equality Duty.
3. Staff should be trained in disability awareness issues and able to offer assistance when it is needed.
4. Do not rely solely on visual appointment systems, such as LCD scrolling information boards displaying appointments, which cannot be used by people with sight loss.
5. Ensure that medication and prescription information is accessible to blind and partially sighted people by using new systems, such as x-pil, which implement an EU Directive, and community pharmacist programmes.

It is clear that print format is not necessarily the first choice of information source for people with visual impairment; however, it can still be very useful. The RNIB have a number of guidelines for written information that are based on consultation and research.

PRINT GUIDELINES
- Type size: the RNIB recommend a type size between 12 point and 14 point.
- Contrast is important and the better the contrast, the more accessible the information will be. Black text on a white background provides best contrast.
- Typeface should be plain, and a typeface should be chosen in which numbers are very clear – 3 and 5 and 8 and 0 are often confused.
- Type styles: blocks of capital letters are very difficult to read. Odd words in capital letters are fine but large areas should be avoided. Underlined words or italics are also very difficult and

text should be highlighted in other ways such as the use of bold.

- Line spacing: for optimum contrast, line spacing should be 1.5–2.
- Type weight: people with visual problems often prefer bold or semi-bold weights to normal ones.
- Word spacing and alignment: text should be aligned to the left margin only. Justified text should be avoided because it changes the spaces between letters and words, which makes reading more difficult.
- Columns: a large space should separate columns to make them obvious. If space is limited, a vertical line should be drawn between the columns.
- Setting text: unless all lines still start at the same place, fitting text around images should be avoided. Text on top of images or texture should also be avoided because contrast is reduced.
- Forms: more space on forms is needed because people with partial sight tend to have larger handwriting.
- Paragraphs: a space should be left between paragraphs to break up the page and make section breaks more obvious.
- Navigation: page numbers and heading should be in the same place to aid navigation around the document.
- Printing: glossy paper should be avoided because glare makes reading more difficult. The paper should be heavy enough that text does not show through from the other side.

More information can be obtained from seeitright@rnib.org.uk

EMAIL
Email can be a very useful information-giving tool for people with visual disability. Text can be increased in size to a point where it is legible for the individual. If patients wish to have information such as appointments sent by email, this service should be available to them.

WEB INFORMATION
Web information is relied on by many people who are blind or have visual impairment. Reading programs mean that the

internet is accessible to those with very little or no vision and the world of information is available, provided that websites are of a high standard. The RNIB also publishes guidelines on web accessibility and undertakes audit, awarding a logo to those sites that achieve the audit standards.

The law is also an issue here and it has been a legal requirement for UK websites to be accessible since 1999.

REFERENCE

Royal National Institute for the Blind (2007). *Information is Power*. London: RNIB. Available at: www.rnib.org.uk/xpedio/groups/public/documents/publicwebsite/public_infopower.hcsp (accessed 30 May 2007).

New pathways for common eye conditions

The Eye Care Services Steering Group within the Department of Health (DH) has done a considerable amount of work on revisions to and recommendations for streamlined pathways for four common eye problems: cataract, glaucoma, age-related macular degeneration (AMD) and low vision (DH 2004)

The glaucoma, AMD and low vision pathways were piloted with varying degrees of success (McLeod et al. 2006). The cataract pathway was based on existing good practice and *Action on Cataracts* (DH 2000).

Cataract pathway

The pathway in Figure 63.1 follows the recommendations in *Action on Cataracts* (DH 2000), which are in place, and adapted in most ophthalmic units in England and the wider UK.

The suggested pathways for the other conditions are built on expertise of clinicians, service users and user groups and policy-makers in an attempt to streamline pathways for these conditions and achieve equity across the ophthalmic sector.

Proposed glaucoma pathway (DH 2004)

The pathway in Figure 63.2 shows an enhanced role for the community optometrist and the need for an increasing number of optometrists with a special interest (OSI) in glaucoma and ophthalmic medical practitioners (OMPs) in the community. It also suggests an extra stage in the process: instead of optometrists referring to the hospital eye service (HES), the patient is referred to an OMP or OSI, who makes the diagnosis and starts treatment, or refers on to the HES. It also shows a much greater reliance on the optometrist to manage patients with glaucoma in the community.

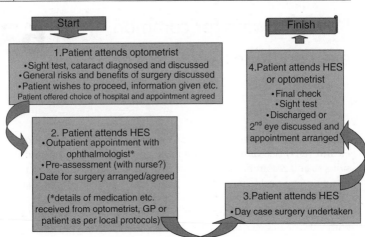

Figure 63.1 Cataract pathway (DH 2000). HES, hospital eye service.

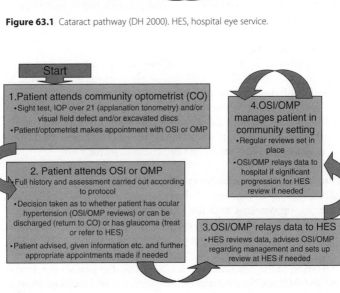

Figure 63.2 Proposed glaucoma pathway (DH 2004). CO, community optometrist; HES, hospital eye service; OMP, ophthalmic medical practitioner; OSI, optometrist with a special interest in glaucoma.

63

Proposed AMD pathway (DH 2004)

The pathway in Figure 63.3 again relies heavily on the patient attending an OSI in AMD. If the patient presents to an optometrist without specialist knowledge of AMD, rather than add an extra step of an appointment with an OSI, it might be felt that the patient would be better referred to the HES to save time in the case of treatable 'wet' AMD. It does recognise that many patients with 'dry' AMD are not treatable and need timely information and access to rehabilitation and other services.

Proposed low vision pathway (DH 2004)

The pathway in Figure 63.4 recognises the fragmented nature of low vision services and attempts to show a pathway that could be adopted as a standard (see also Chapter 59, Recommendations for low vision services).

The three pathways in Figures 63.2–63.4 were piloted in a number of different centres, using different formats across

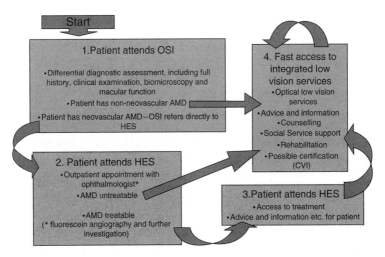

Figure 63.3 Proposed age-related macular degeneration (AMD) pathway. CVI, Certificate of Vision Impairment; HES, hospital eye service; OSI, optometrist with a special interest in AMD.

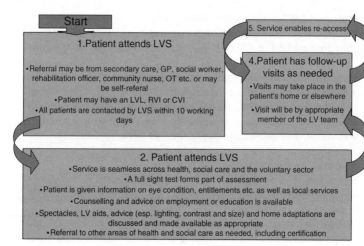

Figure 63.4 Proposed low vision pathway. CVI, Certificate of Vision Impairment; LV, low vision; LVL, Low Vision Leaflet; LVS, low vision service; RVI, Referral of Vision Impairment.

England, and the evaluation group reported in 2006 (McLeod et al. 2006).

Key points from the pilots included the following:

- Change is difficult and takes time to implement. It is particularly challenging when working across boundaries such as those of primary and secondary care, and when incorporating health care, social care and the third sector (the 'voluntary' sector).
- Strong relationships are needed between partners in order to improve service delivery. Relationships initially are often personal rather than organisationally led.
- Mapping of current service delivery, and considering future demand, capacity issues, patient engagement and cost–benefit analysis, must all be considered during the process of service re-design.
- Communication strategies are vital to ensure engagement of stakeholders.

63

- New ways of working should respond to local need and circumstances. There is no 'one-size-fits-all' model.
- Voluntary sector organisations are often the most appropriate to take the leading role in low vision services.
- Patients particularly like new schemes for glaucoma and low vision management.
- Community-based services can significantly reduce travelling time for patients.
- A critical success factor in co-management of glaucoma using an optometrist is an effective partnership with consultant ophthalmologists, which is achieved more easily if they lead the process.
- A significant number of false positives for wet ARMD were encountered in the ARMD pathway pilots. This required the development of a fast-track clinic (in the pilots, led by a doctor, but, in practice, in other centres, this may be nurse led) to confirm diagnosis.
- Rapid assessment of patients with suspected wet ARMD remains an important challenge.
- Training, audit and skills maintenance are critical issues in services, including all new services, and should be in place from the outset.

All these pathways aim to achieve more timely care for the ever-increasing number of patients with chronic eye conditions and have major lessons for the organisation of ophthalmic services and the partnerships that they can achieve with other health-care and social care providers and the third sector.

REFERENCES

Department of Health (2000). *Action on Cataracts*. London: DH.
Department of Health (2004). *First Report of the National Eye Care Services Steering Group*. London: DH.
McLeod H, Dickinson H, Williams I, Robinson S, Coast J (2006). *Evaluation of the Chronic Eye Care Services Programme: Final report*. Health Services Management Centre, University of Birmingham.

The Disability Discrimination Act

The Disability Discrimination Act (DDA) 1995 aimed to end the discrimination that many disabled people face. This Act gave disabled people rights in the areas of:

- employment
- education
- access to goods, facilities and services
- buying or renting land or property.

The Act also allows the Government to set minimum standards so that disabled people can use public transport easily.

In April 2005 a new Disability Discrimination Act was passed by Parliament, which amended or extended existing provisions in the DDA 1995, including:

- making it unlawful for operators of transport vehicles to discriminate against disabled people
- making it easier for disabled people to rent property and for tenants to make disability-related adaptations
- making sure that private clubs with 25 or more members cannot keep disabled people out, just because they have a disability
- extending protection to cover people who have HIV, cancer and multiple sclerosis from the moment that they are diagnosed
- ensuring that discrimination law covers all the activities of the public sector
- requiring public bodies to promote equality of opportunity for disabled people.

The final sections of the Act came into force in January 2006.

The development of legislation to improve the rights of disabled people is an ongoing process. From 1 October 2004, Part 3 of the DDA 1995 has required businesses and other organisations to take reasonable steps to tackle physical features that act as a barrier to disabled people who want to access their services.

This may mean removing, altering or providing a reasonable means of avoiding physical features of a building that make access impossible or unreasonably difficult for disabled people. Examples include:

- putting in ramps
- providing larger, well-defined signs for people with a visual impairment
- improving access to toilet and washing facilities.

The Act places a duty on the public sector to promote equality of opportunity for disabled people and to eliminate all discrimination. All public authorities must review their policies, practices, procedures and services to make sure that they do not discriminate against disabled people and ensure that all their services are planned with disabled people's needs fully considered in advance. Public bodies will have to produce Action Plans on how they intend to meet their duties and review their progress annually.

All disabled people have a right to information about health care and Social Services in a format that is accessible to them. This should include the production of appointment and information letters and leaflets in large print, or even Braille to assist those with visual impairment.

Ophthalmic services need to be creative about solutions to problems such as appointment letters and recognise that many people with visual impairment use technological solutions to minimise the impact of their disability. Facilities such as texts to mobile phones, and particularly email, can be very useful for visually impaired people. Many have computers that read their emails to them, or are able to exchange font size to make the words more readable. In this way, visually impaired people are not disadvantaged by receiving communications that they cannot read.

THE DISABILITY RIGHTS COMMISSION (DRC)

The Disability Rights Commission (DRC) was set up by the Government to help secure civil rights for disabled people and produces guidance and further information on the law and disability.

The DRC helpline provides advice and information about the DDA 1995 to disabled people, employers, service providers, schools and colleges, and friends and families of disabled people:

Telephone: 0845 762 2633
Textphone: 0845 762 2644
Fax: 0845 777 8878
See also www.direct.gov.uk/en/DisabledPeople/index.htm

64

FURTHER INFORMATION

Disability Discrimination Act 1995: www.opsi.gov.uk/acts/acts1995/1995050.htm

Disability Discrimination Act 2005: www.opsi.gov.uk/ACTS/acts2005/20050013.htm

Explanatory notes to the Disability Discrimination Act 2005: www.opsi.gov.uk/ACTS/en2005/2005en13.htm

Visual health and Government priorities

Government policy affects health priorities. Table 65.1 shows some of the current policy issues and how they link to visual health. These may be of great use when formulating business cases or in forming links and partnerships with other health-care and social care sectors.

Table 65.1 Government policy

Older People's National Service Framework (NSF) (DH 2001b)	Standard 2: Person Centred Care Standard 5: Stroke: can give rise to significant vision problems such as hemianopia and quadrantanopia Cranial nerve palsies can give diplopia Standard 6: Falls: there is evidence to suggest a link between visual impairment and falls. There is also some evidence to suggest that older people from lower socioeconomic groups are less likely to access services and there may be unmet need in these groups Standard 7: Mental Health in Older People: vision loss is linked to depression Standard 8: The Promotion of Health and Active Life in Old Age
Children's NSF (DH 2004b)	Standard 1: Children, Young People and Maternity Services The NSF deals with the need to promote the health and well-being of children and young people, identifying needs and intervening early in order to maximise the long-term gain. This standard highlighted the need for a national, orthoptist-led pre-school vision screening programme
Choosing Health	Recent public health initiatives such as *Choosing Health* and *Health Challenge England* (DH 2004a, 2006) have focused on public health problems such as obesity, nutrition and smoking-related illness. ARMD is strongly linked to smoking, with a weak link to nutrition. Obesity is strongly linked to the development of type 2 diabetes
Diabetes NSF (DH 2001a)	The diabetes NSF introduced screening for diabetic retinopathy in adults with diabetes and early laser treatment for those identified as having sight-threatening retinopathy The NSF also introduced a standard to improve detection of diabetes, which can help to prevent retinopathy

REFERENCES

Department of Health (2001a). *National Service Framework for Diabetes*. London: DH.

Department of Health (2001b). *A National Service Framework for Older People*. London: DH.

Department of Health (2004a). *Choosing Health: Making health choices easier*. London: DH.

Department of Health (2004b). *National Service Framework for Children, Young People and Maternity Services*. London: DH.

Department of Health (2006). *Health Challenge England – Next Steps for Choosing Health*. London: DH.

65

Appendices

Appendix 1

Orthoptic abbreviations

ACS	alternating convergent squint
ADS	alternating divergent squint
AHP	abnormal head posture
ARC	abnormal retinal correspondence
BD	base down
BE	both eyes
BEO	both eyes open
BI	base in
BO	base out
BSV	binocular single vision
BT or BTXA	botulinum toxin
BU	base up
BV	binocular vision
BVA	binocular visual acuity
CC or CAC	Cardiff acuity cards (vision test for babies)
CI	convergence insufficiency
c/o	complains of
Conv	convergence/convergent
CPEO	chronic progressive external ophthalmoplegia
CT	cover test
D	dioptre
Dep	depression
Dist	distance
Div	divergence/divergent
DVD	dissociated vertical deviation
DVM	delayed visual maturation
EE	either eye
EF	eccentric fixation
Elev	elevation

Eso	esotropia/-phoria
Exo	exotropia/-phoria
FCPL	forced choice preferential looking (vision test for babies)
FEE	fixing either eye
FLE	fixing left eye
FRE	fixing right eye
FTTO	full time total occlusion
H/A	headache
HES(1)	hospital eye service prescription
HM	hand movements
INO	internuclear ophthalmoplegia
IO	inferior oblique
IR	inferior rectus
Kay Pics	Kay pictures (vision test for children)
LCS	left convergent squint
LDS	left divergent squint
LE	left eye
LPS	levator palpebrae superioris
LR	lateral rectus
L/R	left over right (left hypertropia/-phoria or right hypotropia/-phoria)
LVA	low visual aid or left visual acuity
MR	medial rectus
N	nerve
NAD	no apparent deviation
NPA	near point of accommodation
NPC	near point of convergence
NPL	no perception of light
NRC	normal retinal correspondence
NVA	near visual acuity
o/a	over-action
OKN	optokinetic nystagmus
OM	ocular movements
PBD	prism base down
PBI	prism base in
PBO	prism base out
PBU	prism base up

PCT	prism cover test
PFR	prism fusion range
PH	pinhole
PL	perception of light
PMT	post-mydriatic test
PRT	prism reflection test
PTTO	part time total occlusion
RAF	Royal Air Force rule measurement of convergence and accommodation
RAPD	relative afferent pupillary defect
RCS	right convergent squint
RDS	right divergent squint
Recess	recession
Resect	resection
R/L	right over left (right hypertropia/-phoria or left hypotropia/-phoria)
ROP	retinopathy of prematurity
rr	rapid recovery (as in latent deviations)
RVA	right visual acuity
SG or SSG	single Sheridan Gardiner (vision test for children)
Sl rec	slow recovery (as in latent deviations)
Sn	Snellen
SO	superior oblique
SP	simultaneous perception
SR	superior rectus
u/a	under-action
VA	visual acuity
VEP	visual evoked potential
VER	visual evoked response
VF	visual field
VOR	vestibular ocular reflex

Appexdix 1

Appendix 2

Glossary

Accommodation: the adjustment of the eye for seeing at near distances. The shape of the lens is changed through action of the ciliary muscle, focusing a clear image on the retina.

Achromatopsia: colour blindness.

Agnosia: the inability to recognise common objects despite an intact visual apparatus, for example, prosopagnosia – the inability to recognise faces.

Amaurosis fugax: transient loss of vision, often caused by carotid artery disease.

Amblyopia: reduced visual acuity (uncorrectable) in the absence of detectable anatomical defect in the eye or visual pathways.

Ammetropia: an optical defect preventing light rays from being brought to a focus on the retina.

Amsler grid: a chart with vertical and horizontal lines and a central spot, used in the assessment of macular disease.

Angiography: a diagnostic test in which the retinal vascular system is examined. Intravenous injection of fluorescein demonstrates the retinal circulation, or of indocyanine green demonstrates the choroidal circulation.

Aniridia: congenital absence of the iris.

Anisocoria: unequal pupillary size.

Anisometropia: difference in refractive error of the eyes.

Anophthalmos: absence of a true eyeball.

Aphakia: absence of the lens.

Asthenopia: eye fatigue from muscular, environmental or psychological causes.

Astigmatism: refractive error preventing the light rays from coming to a focus on the retina because of different curvatures of the meridians of the cornea (or lens).

Binocular vision: ability of the eyes to focus on one object and then to fuse the two images into one.

Bitot's spots: keratinisation of the conjunctiva near the limbus, resulting in raised spots – caused by vitamin A deficiency.

Blepharitis: inflammation of the lid margins.

Blepharoptosis: drooping of the eyelid, usually known as ptosis.

Blepharospasm: involuntary spasm of the eyelids.

Blind spot: missing area of the visual field, corresponding to where light falls on the optic nerve head.

Botulinum toxin: neurotoxin A of the bacterium *Clostridium botulinum* used in very small doses to produce temporary paralysis of the extraocular muscles.

Buphthalmos: large eyeball in congenital glaucoma caused by raised pressure.

Canthotomy: usually a lateral canthotomy cutting of the lateral canthal tendon in order to widen the palpebral fissure. Commonly after trauma because of haematoma in the orbit.

Canthus: the angle formed at the junction of the upper and lower lids – inner (medial) and outer (lateral).

Capsulorrhexis: removal of the anterior capsule of the lens before phakoemulsification, using a single, circular tear.

Capsulotomy (posterior): laser treatment after 'extracapsular cataract extraction' involving the making of a hole in the posterior capsule of the lens that has become opaque.

Cartella: protective eye shield.

Chalazion: swelling of a meibomian gland as a result of infection or granuloma after an infection.

Chemosis: conjunctival oedema.

Coloboma: congenital cleft in ocular tissue caused by the failure of a part of the eye or adnexae to form completely.

Concave lens: lens with the power to diverge rays of light; also known as diverging or minus lens (–).

Cones: retinal receptor cells, concerned with visual acuity and colour discrimination.

Convex lens: lens with the power to converge rays of light and to bring them into focus on the retina.

Cyclitis: inflammation of the ciliary body.

Cyclodestructive procedures: surgical techniques to reduce aqueous production by destroying part of the ciliary body using cryotherapy (cyclocryotherapy), lasers (cyclophotoco-agulation) or diathermy.

Cycloplegic: a drug that temporarily paralyses the ciliary muscle.

Cylindrical lens: a segment of a cylinder (the refractive power of which varies in different meridians) used to correct astigmatism.

Dacryoadenitis: infection of the lacrimal gland.

Dacryocystitis: infection of the lacrimal sac.

Dacryocystorhinostomy: a procedure by which a channel is made between the nasolacrimal duct and the nasal cavity to bypass an obstruction in the nasolacrimal duct or sac.

Dark adaptation: the ability to adjust to decreased illumination.

Dellen: an area of epithelial loss on the cornea caused by drying as a result of shadowing by a conjunctiva swollen by chemosis or subconjunctival haemorrhage.

Dendritic ulcer: a corneal ulcer caused by herpes simplex virus – named thus because of the characteristic pattern of the ulcer on the cornea.

Dioptre: unit of measurement of the refractive power of lenses.

Diplopia: double vision – the eye's inability to fuse two images into one – disappears when one eye is covered.

Discission: operation for congenital cataract or certain types of traumatic cataract in which the anterior capsule is ruptured and the lens substance left to absorb or, later, be evacuated.

Ecchymosis: 'black eye'.

Ectropion: turning out of the eyelid (eversion).

Emmetropia: an eye with no refractive error.

Endolaser: application of laser from a probe inside the globe.

Endophthalmitis: intraocular infection.

Enophthalmos: abnormal retrodisplacement of the eyeball.

Entropion: a condition where the eyelid turns inward (inversion).

Enucleation: surgical removal of the eyeball.

Epicanthus: congenital skin fold that overlies the inner canthus.

Epiphora: watering eye – tearing.

Evisceration: removal of the contents of the globe.

Exenteration: removal of the entire contents of the orbit, including the globe and lids. May be more or less radical.

Exophthalmos: abnormal protrusion of the eyeball (proptosis).

Field of vision: the entire area that can be seen without moving the point of gaze.

Floaters: moving images in the visual field caused by vitreous opacities.

Fornix: the junction of the bulbar and palpebral conjunctivae.

Fovea: depression in the macula adapted for most acute vision.

Fundus: the posterior portion of the eye visible through an ophthalmoscope.

Glaucomaflecken: opacities on the anterior lens capsule indicative of a previous episode of acute angle-closure glaucoma.

Gonioscopy: an examination technique for the anterior chamber angle, using a corneal contact lens containing a mirror and a light source.

Hemianopia: blindness in one-half of the field of vision of one or both eyes (bitemporal, where both temporal fields are missing, or homonymous, where the defect is on the same side).

Hippus: spontaneous rhythmic movements of the iris.

Hordeolum, external (stye): infection of the glands of Moll or Zeiss.

Hordeolum, internal: meibomian gland infection – chalazion.

Hypermetropia (farsightedness): a refractive error in which the focus of light from a distant object is behind the retina.

Hyphaema: blood in the anterior chamber.

Hypopyon: pus in the anterior chamber.

Hypotony: abnormally soft eye from any cause.

Injection: congestion of blood vessels.

Iridodialysis: detachment of the iris from the ciliary body, caused usually by blunt trauma.

Iridodonesis: trembling of the iris after cataract extraction.

Ishihara colour plates: a test for colour vision based on the ability to see patterns in a series of multicoloured charts.

Isopter: an object for testing visual fields. Isopters can be of different colours and sizes, and form concentric rings on field testing (perimetry).

Keratic precipitate: accumulation of inflammatory cells on the corneal endothelium in uveitis.

Keratitis: corneal inflammation.

Keratoconus: cone-shaped deformity of the cornea.

Keratomalacia: corneal softening, usually associated with vitamin A deficiency.

Keratometer: an instrument for measuring the curvature of the cornea.

Keratoplasty: corneal graft – may be lamellar or full thickness. An area of opaque cornea is replaced in order to achieve corneal clarity.

Keratotomy: an incision in the cornea. Radial keratotomy is a procedure in which radial incisions are made in the cornea to change the curvature of the cornea and correct refractive error.

Leukocoria: white pupil.

Limbus: junction of the cornea and sclera.

Macula lutea: the small avascular area of the retina surrounding the fovea, containing yellow xanthophyll pigment.

Megalocornea: abnormally large cornea.

Metamorphopsia: distortion of vision.

Microphthalmos: abnormally small eye with abnormal function.

Miotic: a drug causing pupillary constriction.

Mydriatic: a drug causing pupillary dilatation.

Myopia (nearsightedness): a refractive error in which the focus for light rays from a distant object is in front of the retina, so images from a distance appear blurred.

Nanophthalmos: abnormally small eye with normal function.

Near point: the point at which the eye is focused when accommodation is fully active.

Nystagmus: an involuntary movement of the globe that may be horizontal, vertical, torsional or mixed.

Ophthalmia neonatorum: conjunctivitis in the newborn.

Optic disc: ophthalmoscopically visible portion of the optic nerve.

Pannus: infiltration of the cornea with blood vessels.

Panophthalmitis: inflammation of the entire globe.

Papillitis: optic nerve head inflammation.

Perimeter: an instrument for measuring the visual field.

Peripheral vision: ability to perceive the presence or motion of objects outside the direct line of vision.

Phakoemulsification: technique of extracapsular cataract extraction in which the nucleus of the lens is disrupted into small fragments by ultrasonic vibrations, allowing aspiration of lens matter through a small wound, leading to faster visual recovery.

Phlycten: localised lymphocytic infiltration of the conjunctiva or corneal margin, resulting in a small, raised, staining area.

Photocoagulation: thermal damage to tissues, in ophthalmology, usually as a result of laser energy.

Photophobia: abnormal sensitivity to light.

Photopsia: appearance of flashes of light within the eye caused by traction on the retina.

Phthisis bulbi: atrophy of the globe with blindness and decreased intraocular pressure, caused by end-stage ophthalmic disease.

Pinguecula: a thickening of the conjunctiva, usually medial to the cornea; bilateral and a normal finding.

Placido's disc: a disc with concentric black and white rings used to determine the regularity of the cornea by observing the ring's reflection on the corneal surface.

Presbyopia: physiologically blurred near vision, caused by reduction in the ability of the eye to accommodate, as a result of increasing size and rigidity of the lens with age.

Pseudophakia: presence of an artificial intraocular lens after cataract extraction.

Pterygium: a triangular growth of tissue that extends from the conjunctiva over the cornea.

Ptosis: drooping of the eyelid.

Puncta: external orifices of the upper and lower canaliculi.

Refraction: (a) deviation in the course of light rays passing from one transparent medium into another of different density; (b) determination of refractive errors of the eye.

Appexdix 2

Retinal detachment: a separation of the neurosensory retina from the pigment epithelium.

Retinitis pigmentosa: a hereditary degeneration of the retina.

Retinoscope: an instrument designed for objective refraction of the eye.

Rods: retinal receptor cells concerned with peripheral vision and vision in decreased illumination.

Rubeosis: aberrant blood vessels, often on the iris (rubeosis iridis).

Scleral spur: the protrusion of sclera into the anterior chamber angle.

Scotoma: a blind or partially blind area in the visual field.

Staphyloma: a thinned part of the coat of the eye resulting in protrusion of ocular contents.

Strabismus: misalignment of the eyes – a squint.

Subconjunctival haemorrhage: haemorrhage, generally idiopathic, underneath the conjunctiva.

Symblepharon: adhesions between the bulbar and palpebral conjunctivae.

Sympathetic ophthalmia: inflammation in a normal eye resulting from inflammation in the fellow eye.

Synechiae: adhesion of the iris to the cornea (anterior synechiae) or lens (posterior synechiae).

Syneresis: a degenerative process within the vitreous involving a drawing together of particles within the gel, separation and shrinkage of the gel.

Tarsorrhaphy: a surgical procedure by which the upper and lower lid margins are joined.

Tonometer: an instrument for measuring intraocular pressure.

Trabeculectomy: surgical procedure for creating a channel for additional aqueous drainage in glaucoma.

Trabeculoplasty: laser photocoagulation of the trabecular meshwork to aid aqueous outflow.

Trachoma: a serious form of infectious keratoconjunctivitis.

Trichiasis: inversion and rubbing of the eyelashes against the globe.

Uveal tract: the iris, ciliary body and choroid.

Uveitis: inflammation of one or all portions of the uveal tract.

Appendix 2

Visual acuity: measure of the central vision.

Visual axis: a theoretical line connecting a fixation point with the fovea centralis.

Vitritis: inflammation of vitreous.

Xerosis: drying of tissues lining the anterior surface of the eye.

Zonule: the suspensory ligaments that stretch from the ciliary processes to the lens equator and hold it in place.

Appendix 3

Useful addresses

International Resource Centre (IRC)
International Centre for Eye Health (ICEH), London School of
  Hygiene and Tropical Medicine, Keppel Street, London WC1E
  7HT, UK
Website: www.iceh.org.uk
Healthlink Worldwide
Cityside, 40 Adler Street, London E1 1EE, UK
Website: www.healthlink.org.uk
Teaching Aids at Low Cost (TALC)
PO Box 49, St Albans, Herts, UK
Website: www.talcuk.org
Christian Blind Mission International (CBMI)
Nibelungenstrasse 124, 64625 Bensheim, Germany
Website: www.cbmi.org
ORBIS International Inc.
520 Eighth Avenue, 11th Floor, New York, NY 10080, USA
Website: www.orbis.org

ORBIS exists to preserve and restore sight worldwide. We
work in partnership with local health professionals to
improve the quality of eye care available for people in countries where the need is great.

Sight Savers International
Grosvenor Hall, Bolnore Road, Haywards Heath, W. Sussex
  RH16 4BX, UK
Website: www.sightsavers.org.uk

VISION 2020 – London Office

London School of Hygiene and Tropical Medicine, Keppel Street, London WC1E 7HT, UK

Website: www.v2020.org

Vision Aid Overseas (VAO)

12 The Bell Centre, Newton Road, Manor Royal, Crawley RH10 2FZ, UK

Website: www.vao.org.uk

World Health Organization (WHO)

Prevention of Blindness and Deafness (PBD), 1211 Geneva 27, Switzerland

Website: www.who.int/pbd

International Agency for the Prevention of Blindness (IAPB)

VISION 2020 – Central Office/IAPB Secretariat, L.V. Prasad Eye Institute, L.V. Prasad Marg, Banjara Hills, Hyderabad, India

Website: www.iapb.org

Global Vision

Website: www.global-vision.org.uk

> . . . is a charitable organisation dedicated to the relief of blindness in developing countries. . . . in the designated country, the eye clinics can be run by Global Vision's volunteer optometrists

SPECS

Website: www.eyeconditions.org.uk

> SPECS is a not-for-profit organisation that provides support to a wide range of organisations dedicated to . . . reviews of UK WWW sites related to the eye, vision and ophthalmology . . .

EyeUK

Website: www.eyeuk.com

> Links to and reviews of UK WWW sites related to the eye, vision and ophthalmology. EyeUK is a non-commercial WWW site with the sole aim of promoting UK Internet access to information on the eye, vision . . . .

EQUIP – Electronic Quality Information for Patients
Website: www.equip.nhs.uk/topics/eye.html

A gateway to quality-checked websites of information for patients.

Action for Blind People
Website: www.afbp.org

Action for Blind People enables blind and partially sighted people to transform their lives through work, housing, leisure and support. We offer a wide range of services to visually impaired people, their families, advocates, professionals and the general public.

Diabetes UK
Website: www.diabetes.org.uk

Diabetes UK is the leading charity working for people with diabetes.

British Blind Sport
Website: www.britishblindsport.org.uk/
British Blind Golf Association
Website: www.blindgolf.co.uk/index.php

The EBGA is a voluntarily run organisation, which provides quality competition and training in golf for registered blind people throughout England and Wales.

The Guide Dogs for the Blind Association
Website: www.guidedogs.org.uk
The Royal College of Ophthalmologists
17 Cornwall Terrace, London NW1 4QW
Tel: +44 (0) 20 7935 0702
Fax: +44 (0) 20 7935 9838
Website: www.rcophth.ac.uk
The Eyecare Trust
Website: www.eyecare-trust.org.uk

The Eyecare Trust is a registered charity that exists to raise awareness of all aspects of ocular health, the importance of regular eye care and good eye wear. We do this by providing accurate, unbiased eye care information to the public and the media.

St John Eye Hospital
Nablus Road, Sheikh Jarrah, Jerusalem 97200, Israel
Website: www.stjohneyehospital.org
Eye Cancer Network
Website: www.eyecancer.com

Provides education and services to patients and professionals.

Positive Vision
Website: www.positivevision.co.uk

Charity that aims to help people with sight loss and to help their families and carers.

Sense
Website: www.sense.org.uk

A voluntary organisation working with people of all ages who are deafblind or have associated disabilities.

Eyetext
Website: www.eyetext.net

Eyetext is an interactive ophthalmology site.

Ophthalmic Hyperguide
Website: www.ophthalmic.hyperguides.com

Educational resource for eye care specialists.

Anaesthesia for ENT, Ophthalmic, Dental and Facial Surgery
The Virtual Anaesthesia Textbook
Website: www.virtual-anaesthesia-textbook.com/vat/ent.html
Eyesite
Website: www.nurseseyesite.nhs.uk

An on-line community for ophthalmic nurses.

The International Council of Ophthalmology
Website: www.icoph.org

The International Council of Ophthalmology's Eye Site is a guide to finding information, resources and connections related to ophthalmology and vision around the world.

It offers information on ophthalmological organisations, ophthalmic education, the preservation and restoration of vision, and the prevention of blindness.

The Eye Site is also the internet home for the International Federation of Ophthalmological Societies (IFOS) and the International Council of Ophthalmology (ICO).

National Radiological Protection Board (NRPB)
Chilton, Didcot, Oxford OX11 0RQ, UK
Website: www.nrpb.org.uk
Unite for Sight
Website: www.uniteforsight.org

Unite for Sight is a non-profit organisation that empowers communities worldwide to improve eye health and eliminate preventable blindness. Local and visiting volunteers work with partner eye clinics to provide eye care in communities without previous access, with the goal of creating eye disease-free communities.

The Thomas Pocklington Trust
Website: www.pocklington-trust.org.uk

UK charity providing housing, care and support services for people with sight loss. They have a good range of research publications around life with sight loss.

St Dunstan's
Website: www.st-dunstans.org.uk

St Dunstan's was established in 1915. When men blinded in combat started coming back from the First World War it was decided that a hostel should be opened for these soldiers and sailors with the vision that, given training, they could be transformed from recipients of charity to people who could lead independent, useful and satisfying lives. In 2000 St Dunstan's extended its services to include those who had

Appexdix 3

served their country and became visually impaired through an accident, illness or age. St Dunstan's continues to help all its members to achieve independent, fulfilling and meaningful lives after blindness.

The Childhood Eye Cancer Trust (CHECT)
Website: www.chect.org.uk

A UK-wide charity for families and individuals affected by retinoblastoma.

The International Glaucoma Association
Website: www.glaucoma-association.com

The International Glaucoma Association (IGA) offers advice and support by sending free patient literature and responding to hundreds of concerns and queries from sufferers every week. The IGA also creates greater public awareness of glaucoma and campaigns for improved glaucoma services. Furthermore it supports considerable clinical research into the nature and treatment of the disease. The IGA encourages early screening for glaucoma, especially those who are particularly at risk because they have relatives with this condition.

The Royal National Institute for the Blind (RNIB)
Website: www.rnib.org.uk
The National Eye Research Centre
Website: www.nerc.co.uk

The NERC is a leading eye charity funding research into some of the most prevalent degenerative and disabling eye conditions. Our research is principally within the University of Bristol, but also in Yorkshire and in other eye centres throughout the UK.

Appendix 4

Useful references and documents

Assistant Directors of Social Services (2002). *Progress in Sight – National Care Standards of Social Care for Visually Impaired Adults*. London: ADSS.

Association of Optometrists (2002). *Low Vision Co-Management*. Available at: www.assoc-optometrists.org

Better Regulation Task Force (2000). *Protecting Vulnerable People*. Available at: www.brc.gov.uk

College of Optometrists (2001). *Framework for a Multidisciplinary Approach to Low Vision*. London: College of Optometrists.

Department of Health (2001). *National Service Framework for Older People, Executive Summary*. London: DH.

Department of Health (2003). *National Service Framework for Children, Young People and Maternity Services*. London: DH. Available at: www.dh.gov.uk/en/Publicationsandstatistics/Publications/PublicationsPolicyAndGuidance/DH_40891122003

Department of Health (2004). *Better Health in Old Age*. London: DH.

Department of Health (2004). *First Report of the National Eye Steering Group*. London: DH.

Department of Health (2006). *Our Health, Our Care, Our Say: A new direction for community services*. Available at: www.dh.gov.uk/en/Publicationsandstatistics/Publications/PublicationsPolicyAndGuidance/DH_4127453

Department of Health (2006). *General Optical Services Review*. London: DH. Available at: www.aop.org.uk/1140086102.html

Department of Health (2007). *Commissioning Toolkit for Community Based Eyecare Services*. London: DH. Available at: www.dh.gov.uk/en/Publicationsandstatistics/Publications/PublicationsPolicyAndGuidance/DH_0639782006

Evans BJW, Rowlands G (2004). Correctable visual impairment in older people: a major unmet need. *Ophthal Physiol Opt* **24**:161–80.

Haymes SA, Johnston AW, Heyes AD (2002). Relationship between vision impairment and ability to perform activities of daily living. *Ophthal Physiol Opt* **22**:79–91.

Low Vision Services Consensus Group (1999). *Low Vision Services Recommendations for Future Service Delivery in the UK*. Available at: www.lowvision.org.uk/publications.html

National Patient Safety Agency (NPSA) (2005). *Seven Steps to Patient Safety*. Available at: www.npsa.nhs.uk/health/resources/7steps

O'Hagan G (1998). *A Sharper Focus: Inspection of services for adults who are visually impaired or blind*. London: DH.

Royal College of Ophthalmologists (1998). *The Hospital Eye Service*. London: RCOphth.

Royal College of Ophthalmologists (2003). *Creutzfeldt–Jakob Disease (CJD) and Ophthalmology*. London: RCOphth.

Royal College of Ophthalmologists (2004). *Guidelines for the Management of Open Angle Glaucoma and Ocular Hypertension*. London: RCOphth.

Thomas Pocklington Trust (2005). *Our Vision Too: Improving the access of ethnic minority visually impaired people to appropriate services; building a supported community referral system*. Available at: www. pocklington-trust.org.uk

Wolffsohn JS, Cochrane AL (2000). Design of the low vision quality-of-life questionnaire (LVQOL) and measuring the outcome of low-vision rehabilitation. *Am J Ophthalmol* **130**:793–802.

World Health Organization (2000). *The Right to Sight – The Global Initiative for the Elimination of Avoidable Blindness*. Geneva: WHO. Available at: www.who.int/pbd/en/WHA56.26.pdf2005

Appexdix 4

Index